Ophthaln

N. M. Evans

Consultant Ophthalmic Surgeon,
The Royal Eye Infirmary, Plymouth

Oxford   New York   Tokyo
OXFORD UNIVERSITY PRESS

Oxford University Press, Walton Street, Oxford OX2 6DP

Oxford   New York
Athens   Auckland   Bangkok   Bombay
Calcutta   Cape Town   Dar es Salaam   Delhi
Florence   Hong Kong   Istanbul   Karachi
Kuala Lumpur   Madras   Madrid   Melbourne
Mexico City   Nairobi   Paris   Singapore
Taipei   Tokyo   Toronto
and associated companies in
Berlin   Ibadan

Oxford is a trade mark of Oxford University Press

Published in the United States
by Oxford University Press Inc., New York

First published in hardback 1995
First published in paperback (with corrections) 1996

A catalogue record for this book is available from the British Library

Library of Congress Cataloging in Publication Data
Evans, Nicholas, FCOphth.
Ophthalmology: a clinical guide / N. M. Evans.
p.   cm. — (Oxford medical publications)
Includes bibliographical references and index.
1. Ophthalmology — Handbooks, manuals, etc.   I. Title.
II. Series.
[DNLM: 1. Eye Diseases — diagnosis — handbooks.   2. Eye Diseases —
therapy — handbooks. WW 39 E92o 1995]
RE48.9.E94   1995   617.7 — dc20   94–49517
DNLM/DLC   for Library of Congress
ISBN 0 19 262407 5 (h/b)
ISBN 0 19 2624067 (p/b)

Typeset by Footnote Graphics, Warminster, Wilts
Printed in Great Britain on acid-free paper by
Bookcraft (Bath) Ltd, Midsomer Norton, Avon

Preface

Ophthalmologists in the early years of their training need an introduction to the clinical methods which are particular to the specialty, practical information and guidance in the management of patients, and a framework upon which to build more advanced study. This book has been written to answer these needs in a concise pocket volume which can be kept conveniently to hand for reference on the ward, in clinic or casualty. Introductory chapters describe the techniques of clinical assessment of the eyes and visual system, and the principles, methods and interpretation of special investigations. There follow chapters covering eye diseases systematically, describing the clinical features, differential diagnosis, pathology, and management of all the disorders likely to be seen in clinical practice. The final chapters cover the management of surgical patients, the basics of ophthalmic optics, the ophthalmic use of lasers, and differential diagnosis of presenting symptoms and signs. Each chapter has a reading list of good modern texts for further detailed study.

Particular attention has been given to providing the kind of specific practical information needed to solve clinical problems (such as: how to approach the differential diagnosis and management of anterior uveitis; how to assess retinal detachment; how to select the appropriate antibiotics to treat endophthalmitis). This clinical information is set in the context of underlying pathology, in order to provide an understanding of the scientific logic of current ophthalmological practice.

Pocket-sized introductions to ophthalmology are often rather limited in scope, giving descriptions of eye disorders, but lacking precise clinical guidance; such information must be sought from large reference texts, which are expensive, and to be found on shelves, not in pockets. This volume represents a distillation of clinical experience — mine and that of my own teachers — which I hope will provide the newcomer to ophthalmology with a useful framework of concepts and principles as well as a convenient source of every day clinical reference.

I am grateful to all those from whom I have learned, to whom I gladly give credit for such merit as the book may contain. The responsibility for such defects as may be found is mine.

Plymouth   N.M.E.
October 1994

Contents

Dose schedules are being continually revised and new side-effects recognized. Oxford University Press makes no representation, express or implied, that the drug dosages in this book are correct. For these reasons the reader is strongly urged to consult the drug company's printed instructions before administering any of the drugs recommended in this book.

1
Clinical assessment

Since the ocular tissues can mostly be inspected directly, ophthalmological assessment is based largely on clinical examination and recognition of normal and abnormal signs. The slit-lamp and ophthalmoscope allow detailed examination of the anterior and posterior segments, while visual, ocular motor, and neurological tests provide information about function in more inaccessible parts of the visual system. Special investigations are helpful in diagnosis and management in some circumstances, but most information is gained by informed history taking and careful examination.

History

Presenting complaint

Visual

Poor vision

Distinguish between: blurring and haziness; dimming and darkening; field loss (uniocular or hemianopia); colour loss. Note that unilateral visual loss which is longstanding or of gradual onset may be noticed incidentally, and mistakenly held to be acute. Left homonymous hemianopia may present as difficulty reading a line of print, or as poor sight in left eye.

Diplopia

Distinguish between uniocular and binocular diplopia (by occluding one eye).

Photopsia

Flashing lights are seen as momentary streaks in the periphery in posterior vitreous detachment and as formed, evolving geometric shapes lasting for minutes in migraine.

Floaters

Floaters are caused by opacities in the vitreous (congenital, degenerative, inflammatory, or haemorrhagic), which may be longstanding, or of recent onset. Congenital vitreous opacities are common and benign, and usually noticed only against a plain background. Posterior vitreous detachment causes floaters which may present with variable blurred vision. A retinal tear is associated with a shower of new floaters, as is vitreous haemorrhage due to retinal neovascularization. Posterior uveitis causes floaters of progressively increasing density.

Distortion

Metamorphopsia is distortion of shape (straight lines become wavy or irregular). It is due to macular distortion (by epiretinal membrane), or leakage from a subretinal neovascular membrane. Micropsia is an abnormally small perceived image, usually due to macular elevation by fluid, typically in central serous retinopathy. Binocular distortions of vision occur with ischaemic or toxic cortical damage, and may be induced by drugs.

Pain

Pain or discomfort in or around the eye is common, but is often not easy to localize or attribute to a specific organic cause. It is commonly referred to the eye from adjacent structures in the sensory distribution of the first division of the trigeminal nerve (V_1), particularly the facial sinuses.

Corneal abrasions, foreign bodies and inflammation cause sharp pain, made worse by eye movement. Conjunctivitis produces grittiness, itching, stinging, or burning. Intraocular inflammation causes a dull ache, accompanied by photophobia.

Pain due to orbital inflammation and retrobulbar neuritis is made worse by eye movements. Intracranial pathology and migraine sometimes cause pain that is referred to the eye. Temporal arteritis is usually associated with pain and tenderness around the eye and over the temple, but may present without pain.

Photophobia

Discomfort caused by light accompanies anterior uveitis and keratitis. Photophobia is a feature of retinal cone disorders (achromatopsia, progressive cone dystrophy). It may be a presenting symptom of buphthalmos. Anterior opacities (corneal scar and anterior cortical cataract) reduce visual acuity in direct light by causing glare.

Discharge

Discharge about the eye arises from inflamed or infected conjunctiva or cornea, from the lacrimal gland or the lacrimal sac. Gram stain may show bacteria or fungi, and pus cells, lymphocytes, or eosinophils, suggesting the cause of the inflammation. Watery discharge may be due to

- oversecretion (surface irritation, tear film instability),
- failure of tear drainage (lid malposition or punctal stenosis),
- obstruction (lacrimal sac or nasolacrimal duct).

Previous ocular history

Determine previous visual status, if possible. Previous sight tests, or history of 'weak' or 'lazy' eye, or of squint during childhood or a period of patching, suggest amblyopia.

Anterior uveitis and herpes simplex keratitis are frequently recurrent, and vernal keratoconjunctivitis may vary seasonally.

General medical history

Diabetes is the commonest cause of treatable retinal vasculopathy; all diabetics should have dilated fundus examination at intervals determined by the state of their retinopathy. Connective tissue disorder, granulomatous inflammation, and systemic vasculitis are all frequently associated with inflammatory eye disease. 'Dry eye' is common in rheumatoid arthritis and sarcoid. Retinal vascular occlusion is associated with hypertension, carotid circulation atheroma, arteriosclerosis, haematological and lipid disorder, and Behçet's disease. Thyroid disease is accompanied by keratopathy, ocular motility disorder, and optic neuropathy.

Family history

Many disorders causing visual loss in infancy and childhood have a hereditary basis; ask if anyone in the family has impaired vision. Both myopia and hypermetropia have a strong familial pattern. Concomitant strabismus commonly occurs in children with affected parents or siblings. Primary open angle glaucoma (POAG) has a higher incidence in those with a positive family history.

Drug history

Vortex keratopathy is caused by amiodarone, and sometimes by amodiaquine. Bull's-eye maculopathy is caused by chloroquine, hydroxychloroquine, and phenothiazines. Ethambutol, streptomycin, isoniazid, and chloramphenicol cause a dose-related optic neuropathy. Nystagmus may be caused by CNS depressants, particularly anticonvulsants.

Examination

Notice the patient's general visual and navigational capacity. Look for abnormal head posture or squint, facial abnormality or asymmetry, proptosis, ptosis or other lid abnormality, or heterochromia (irises of different colour); these signs may be overlooked once a detailed examination begins.

Examine the eyes in a darkened room. Inspect the external eyes and lids, and test the pupil reactions for relative afferent pupil defect (RAPD) using a good light source: a pen torch with good batteries will do, but a powerful focal white beam, such as from a halogen bulb transilluminator, is better. Measure visual acuity without refractive correction, followed by corrected and pinhole acuity, and refraction, if uncorrected vision is poor. Next examine the anterior segment with the slit-lamp, and measure the intraocular pressures. If appropriate test the eye movements for ocular motility disorder, and the visual fields. Dilate the pupils with a short-acting mydriatic (e.g. tropicamide) in order to examine the posterior segments with the indirect ophthalmoscope, and at the slit-lamp with a fundus lens.

Vision

Visual acuity

Acuity is a measure of the capacity of the visual system to resolve detail. It is recorded as a fraction according to Snellen notation, using a standard test-type chart at a set distance from the patient, under constant illumination: 6/6, or 1.0, indicates that the smallest detail which can be resolved by the tested eye is the same as can be resolved by a healthy emmetropic eye at 6 m. 6/12, or 0.5, indicates that the tested eye can resolve at 6 m detail which a healthy eye would resolve at 12 m. The steps on a Snellen chart are not linear, and alternative charts (logMAR, or minimum angle of resolution) have theoretical advantages. A pinhole compensates for uncorrected refractive errors. Unaided acuity that can be improved with pinhole indicates that reduced acuity has a refractive cause.

Visual field

The most appropriate technique for measuring the visual field (perimetry) depends on the nature of the suspected pathology. Formal perimetric procedures use either a kinetic (a target of constant size and brightness is moved slowly towards the centre until it is perceived), or a static (the size or brightness of a stationary stimulus is increased until it is seen) routine. Points of equal sensitivity on the field are joined by lines called isopters.

Finger counting in the four quadrants reveals dense hemianopia, or sensory inattention.

Confrontation testing compares the field of the examiner with that of the subject. Use a small white target brought towards the centre from outside the field. Hemianopia can be identified sensitively by moving a small bright-red target slowly across the midline, where it becomes duller or desaturated as it moves into the hemianopic field.

Computerized perimeters (Humphrey, Octopus, Dicon, Henson) are sensitive, flexible, easy to operate, and give an automated display and printout, but are relatively costly. Screening tests present suprathreshold stimuli at different points across the field, recording missed presentations as scotomas. Threshold tests vary the brightness of presented stimuli at each point, to determine the threshold of perception at different points on the field. Both suprathreshold and threshold tests take automatic account of the lower sensitivity of the peripheral than the central field. Computerized perimeters incorporate tests of subject reliability, by checking the blindspot and re-checking previously tested points, and can store results for future comparison and statistical analysis.

Friedmann visual field analyser is a static perimeter. The intensity is adjusted according to the age of the subject, to correspond approximately with predicted normal threshold intensity. The test is quick to carry out and the device is easy to operate. The programme of stimuli is fixed and restricted, and the fields it produces are intended for glaucoma screening. They are not very suitable for glaucoma management or neurological assessment.

Goldmann perimeter can be used as a static (like the Friedmann) or kinetic perimeter. It requires some skill and practice to use effectively, but because of its sensitivity and flexibility, it can be used accurately to plot field defects of any type.

Bjerrum (tangent) screen is a flat black cloth divided by black threads into radial and concentric zones. The screen is fixed on a wall, either 1 or 2 m from the subject, who fixates the central point, while targets of various sizes are presented statically or kinetically in the central visual field. The field chart is labelled to indicate size of target/distance from the screen, in millimetres (e.g. 2/2000 denotes a 2 mm target used at a 2 m screen). The tangent screen is a flexible and sensitive way of measuring central fields, and can be used to probe particular areas of field (arcuate areas in glaucoma, and the vertical midline in posterior pathway lesions), very accurately.

Pupils

The neurology and clinical features of pupil abnormalities are discussed more fully in Chapter 8.

Relative afferent pupil defect (RAPD)

The swinging flashlight test for a relative afferent pupil defect (Marcus–Gunn pupil) detects reduced function in one optic nerve relative to the other. Shine a light alternately from one eye to the other, in a cycle of 1–2 s, watching the illuminated pupil. Equal constriction of each pupil indicates equal optic nerve function. If there is reduced optic nerve conduction from one eye, both pupils constrict *less* when the light is shone into the *affected* eye. The examiner observes the illuminated pupil, and it appears that this dilates when illuminated, while the normal pupil constricts.

- RAPD is **positive** in: optic neuropathy (demyelinating, inflammatory, toxic, ischaemic, neoplastic), advanced glaucoma, retinal detachment, central vessel occlusion.
- RAPD is **negative** in: corneal opacity, cataract, vitreous haemorrhage, macular degeneration, because although the image is degraded, optic nerve function is not reduced.

Motor pupil defects

Anisocoria (unequal pupil size) is present in up to 20 per cent of normal individuals (physiological anisocoria). Pathological anisocoria can be caused by:

- affected pupil dilated   III nerve (parasympathetic) disorder
                                    Adie's myotonic pupil
                                    iris trauma (traumatic mydriasis)
                                    mydriatics
- affected pupil constricted   sympathetic pathology (Horner's syndrome)
                                    miotics
- affected pupil irregular   posterior synaechiae
                                    iris atrophy

Pupil diagnostic tests

First, identify the abnormal pupil: if the anisocoria is greater in the dark, the smaller pupil is abnormal (because it has failed to dilate); if the anisocoria is greater in the light, the larger pupil is defective (because it has failed to constrict).

Pupil tests to diagnose the cause of pupil abnormality are described in Chapter 8, p. 166.

Slit-lamp examination

The slit-lamp is a microscope with controllable slit-beam illumination, which allows stereoscopic examination of a thin optical section of the ocular media. The anterior segment is examined directly, but examination of the posterior segment requires accessory lenses. The eyepieces and objectives can be changed to give variable magnification, and filters and an adjustable aperture allow the intensity and colour (blue filter to provide illumination for fluorescein examination, and green for red-free illumination to increase the contrast of blood vessels) of the beam to be varied. The length of the beam is shown on a scale, enabling precise measurement (e.g. of corneal scars). The illuminating column is coaxial with the microscope, but can be diverted off-axis by loosening a screw on the front of the illuminating arm, for retroillumination and scleral scatter.

Methods of illumination

1. *Focal.* Focal illumination is used for most purposes. The focal point of the illuminated slit coincides with the focal plane of the microscope, providing bright even illumination for inspection of the anterior segment.

2. *Specular.* Angle the microscope and illumination symmetrically either side of a perpendicular to the corneal surface. Focus at high magnification with a narrow illuminating beam on to the corneal endothelium. Endothelial surface irregularities (guttata and cell junctions) are highlighted. With sufficient magnification, and using a special instrument (specular photomicrography), individual endothelial cells can be seen.

3. *Scleral scatter.* De-centre the illuminating arm so that it is focused on the limbus, illuminating the cornea diffusely from the side, while inspecting the centre of the cornea directly. Optical irregularities in the stroma and epithelium are highlighted by increased contrast.

4. *Retroillumination*. Shine the illuminating beam axially through the pupil so that the anterior segment is illuminated by light reflected from the fundus. Iris atrophy, iridectomy, iridotomy, and iris depigmentation show as bright transillumination defects. Some lens opacities, and small traumatic corneal and lens penetrations, are best seen by dilated retroilluminated examination.

5. *Red-free*. The red-free filter renders blood vessels black, increasing the contrast between these and the background. Used in conjunction with an accessory fundus lens red-free illumination is helpful in the examination of retinal vascular disease, e.g. diabetic retinopathy or maculopathy, when microaneurysms and neovascularization are easily seen. Red-free light is also useful in estimating the depth of lesions; retinal pigment epithelium (RPE) reflects red-free light, obscuring masses which are entirely subretinal. When these extend forward through the RPE they absorb the red-free, and the lesions appear darker and more sharply outlined.

Staining

Fluorescein and Rose Bengal stain ocular surface abnormalities and epithelial defects. Fluorescein stains the tear film, and bare stroma devoid of overlying epithelial cover. Rose Bengal stains desiccated or devitalized epithelial cells, and mucus fragments in the tear film.

Accessory slit-lamp lenses

Diagnostic lenses are used to extend the focal range of the slit-lamp, to allow stereoscopic biomicroscopy of the drainage angle, and the posterior segment.

Contact diagnostic lenses

Anaesthetize the cornea and put a drop of 20 per cent hypromellose into the corneal surface of the lens. With the patient in position at the slit-lamp and looking upwards, hold the lower lid gently down. As the lens is placed on to the surface of the eye the patient looks forwards, to bring the cornea and lens into contact.

Three-mirror

The central lens gives a view of the posterior pole, the first mirror (all sides straight) of the equator, the second (two straight and one curved side) of the periphery, and the third mirror (curved edge) shows the ciliary body and drainage angle.

Rodenstock panfundoscope, Volk quadraspheric, area centralis, Mainster

These are complex lenses giving wide-angle three-dimensional views of the fundus, which vary from panoramic to central, and are inverted and less stable than that of the three-mirror.

Gonioprism

The gonioprism is a small lens with one or more mirrors used to inspect the drainage angle.

Non-contact diagnostic lenses

78D and 90D lenses
Small high power lenses used at the slit-lamp to give a magnified (and inverted) three-dimensional image of the fundus. A real image is produced between the lens and the slit-lamp's objective, for inspection by the slit-lamp, in the same way as the 20D lens produces an image for inspection by the indirect ophthalmoscope. Hold the lens between forefinger and thumb close to the subject's cornea, coaxial with the illuminating and inspecting axes of the slit-lamp, and withdraw it slowly until an image appears.

Hruby
This is a strong diverging lens which effectively extends the slit-lamp microscope's focal length to give a smaller erect image of the fundus. It has largely been superseded by the 78D and 90D lenses, which give a more useful image.

Intraocular pressure (IOP)

Applanation tonometer

The Goldman tonometer works by measuring the applied force required to applanate (i.e. to make flat) a given surface area of the cornea. This force is proportional to the IOP when the opposing forces of tear film surface tension and corneoscleral rigidity are equal, and therefore cancel each other out. This equilibrium occurs when an area of 7.3 mm^2 is applanated.

Put topical anaesthetic and fluorescein in the eye to be applanated, and bring the tonometer head into contact with the corneal surface. Adjust the applied force until the two halves of the meniscus image (whose image has been offset by 3.06 mm by a prism) join in a lazy S-shape. At this point the meniscus between the tonometer head and the cornea covers a standard area of π. 1.53^2 = 7.35 mm^2, and the IOP is read from the tonometer scale.

Other tonometric techniques

Perkins
A hand-held applanation tonometer similar to the Goldman in which the applanating prism is weighted with a spring instead of a balance, so that it can be used at any angle. It is useful when the slit-lamp cannot be used, e.g. at the bedside, or in wheelchairbound patients, but it is less accurate than a Goldman.

Pulsair
The most recent non-contact tonometer; this uses a puff of air to applanate, and senses, measures, and displays applanation automatically. It is reasonably portable, and reasonably accurate.

Tonopen, McKay–Marg
The pressure on a central probe is unloaded by increasing corneal pressure on its surrounding collar, as the cornea is touched. IOP is measured and displayed automatically. The Tonopen is highly portable and reasonably accurate.

Ophthalmoscopic examination

The direct ophthalmoscope gives a monocular erect image of the fundus, magnified about × 16 and covering about 10°–15°, or 2–3 disc diameters. The indirect ophthalmoscope gives an inverted stereoscopic image of the fundus of less magnification (about × 5), and a correspondingly wider field (about 30°–40°). Scleral indentation can be used to extend the peripheral view given by the indirect ophthalmoscope to include the ora serrata.

Fundus examination requires dilated pupils. Begin with an overall view, including the periphery, using the indirect. Then inspect the disc, macula, and any abnormalities in detail with the 90D or 78D at the slit-lamp, or the direct ophthalmoscope.

Dilatation

Check that the angles are not dangerously narrow before dilating. Dilate both pupils, so that both fundi can be compared, unless there is a specific contraindication. Tropicamide produces dilatation of short duration (3–6 h) with minimal cycloplegia, and is sufficient for most diagnostic purposes. Supplement tropicamide if necessary using 10 per cent phenylephrine drops.

Indirect ophthalmoscope

Set the inter-pupillary distance (IPD) by adjusting the eyepieces individually so that each eye sees a full rectangular field, superimposed into one when both eyes are open. Adjust the position of the light so that it illuminates just above the centre of the pupil, and its intensity so that a clear view is obtained without dazzling the subject. Hold the condensing lens in thumb and index finger, and steady it by resting the middle finger on the brow over the eye to be examined. Position the lens close to the eye, so that it contains a small erect image of the eye. Then withdraw the lens slowly until a clear inverted image of the fundus appears. The 20D lens is most useful for most purposes in adult eyes. The 28D or 30D is better for examining the shorter eyes of infants and children, and can help give an overall view of the topography of retinal detachments.

First examine the posterior pole, looking for abnormalities of the disc, macula, and vessels. Vascular and inflammatory disorders, the pattern of exudates, and elevated lesions are seen well. Next examine the periphery, particularly during search for retinal breaks and during examination of retinal detachment. Indentation of the periphery is a particularly useful adjunct to indirect ophthalmoscope examination when searching the equatorial and pre-equatorial retina for breaks.

Direct ophthalmoscope

The direct ophthalmoscope's greater magnification permits detailed inspection of the disc, macula, and short segments of retinal vessels.

Retinoscopy

Retinoscopy is the technique used to measure the eye's refraction, by assessing the effect of lenses on the behaviour of an image formed by light reflected from the retina. Practical aspects of retinoscopy and refraction are described in detail in Chapter 13, p. 249.

Retinoscopy is usually performed on the unaccommodated eye. In adults and older children it is usually sufficient to 'fog' the fellow eye by placing a positive lens before it to prevent accommodation, but cycloplegia is necessary for retinoscopic refraction of children under 5. Cyclopentolate 1 per cent × 2 at 15 min intervals, half an hour before refraction, is usually adequate. Atropine 1 per cent ointment t.d.s. for the 3 days preceding the examination ensures complete cycloplegia, but is necessary only in those with very heavy iris pigmentation, or if the instillation of drops induces such terror that it is better avoided near the examination room.

Ocular movements

Eye movements are initiated in the supranuclear centres, assembled in the brainstem gaze centres, and executed by the motor nerves from III, IV, and VI nuclei, driving the extraocular muscles.

Duction is movement in one direction of one eye. Uniocular paresis or restriction produces diplopia and incomitant strabismus, maximal in the direction of action (the field) of the affected muscle.

Versions and vergences are, respectively, movements of the two eyes in the same (conjugate) and in opposite (dysjugate) directions. Disorder in the gaze centres or supranuclear centres produces paresis of conjugate gaze, and midbrain disease causes vergence disorder.

Saccades and pursuits are, respectively, fast and slow conjugate eye movements, originating from the prefrontal and occipital cortex, and projecting to the brainstem gaze centres.

Nystagmus is a cyclically oscillating movement of both (rarely one) eyes.

Strabismus (squint) describes deviation of the visual axis of one eye from the fixation target.

Tests of eye movement are described on p. 175.

Fluorescein angiography

Intravenous injection of 5 ml 10 per cent fluorescein creates a bolus of fluorescence which can be followed photographically as it passes through the ocular circulation. Fundus fluorescein angiography (FFA) is used to outline circulation through the retina and choroid, showing leakage and oedema, masses or defects between sclera and vitreous, and circulation through the optic nerve head. Up to 36 frames are taken using flash passed through a cobalt filter, beginning before the dye reaches the eye, and continuing at intervals initially of 1 s and later at longer intervals up to 15–20 min.

The choroidal vessels fill shortly before the retinal vessels, and the retinal arterial phase can be distinguished from the venous phase. Abnormalities are defined as hyperfluorescent (leakage, staining, or window defect) or hypofluorescent (hypoperfusion or masking by an opaque overlying layer).

Full resuscitation facilities, including intravenous adrenaline and hydrocortisone, and oxygen, must be immediately available when fluorescein angiography is performed, since anaphylactic collapse occasionally follows intravenous injection of fluorescein.

Anterior segment fluorescein angiography can be used to identify disorders of circulation at the limbus, in peripheral corneal disease.

Ultrasound

Ophthalmic diagnostic ultrasound (US) is used to image ocular structures hidden by opacity (e.g. retinal detachment behind cataract or vitreous haemorrhage), and to investigate disease of the orbit (B-mode). It is also used to define the tissue characteristics of an intraocular mass, and make precise measurements of intraocular structures, tumours, and dimensions (A-mode). The frequency of US determines resolution and tissue penetration. Ophthalmic instruments generally use 10 mHz.

A-mode scan (amplitude-mode) displays the sonic reflectivity of the structures encountered by a linear beam in one dimension. It is used to measure axial length for the estimation of intraocular lens power in cataract surgery, and to measure growth and define tissue structure of an intraocular masses. Melanoma attenuates the US signal in linear decay, whereas vascular tumours show multiple echogenic planes.

B-mode (brightness mode) displays the sonic reflectivity of a two-dimensional (plane) beam on a two-dimensional grey scale. An image of the plane of the beam is displayed on the screen, which graphically reproduces the structures in that plane, and can be photographed or recorded. It shows the posterior corneal surface, lens, and retina, as well as any abnormal interface which may be present (vitreous haemorrhage, retinal detachment, tumour surface, and calcification).

A-mode scan is performed directly on to the anaesthetized cornea, as in applanation. B-mode scan is performed through closed lids using coupling gel. Most B-mode scans give a vector A-scan, to define the reflectance characteristics of tissues in an axis defined by the user.

X-ray and CT

It is generally preferable to discuss clinical problems requiring diagnostic radiology with the radiologist, in order to identify the most appropriate investigation. With the increasing availability of CT, many indications for plain radiographs have been superseded by the higher quality information that imaging by CT provides.

Plain X-ray

Following trauma, radio-opaque intraocular foreign body may be identified or excluded on plain films. Plain orbit radiographs demonstrate inequality in size between the orbits, and irregularity or erosion of their walls, due to tumour. Sinus X-rays demonstrate pathological opacification, due to tumour or chronic inflammation, and mucocoele; associated nasopharyngeal disease may also be shown. Increased density of the sphenoids is characteristic of sphenoid ridge meningioma, and patchy differences in density occur in Paget's disease and metastatic tumours.

CT and MRI

CT has largely replaced plain radiography in the investigation of pituitary tumour, optic nerve tumour, and orbit blowout. It is particularly useful for demonstrating soft tissue mass in the orbit, intraocular tumour in children and intraocular foreign body. CT and MRI scans show intracranial pathology very much more clearly than plain radiographs. MRI is particularly useful in demonstrating demyelinating plaques.

Angiography

Carotid angiography has been largely superseded by CT scan, but has an important place in defining intracerebral circulation abnormalities, particularly arteriovenous shunts and in the management of intracranial aneurysms.

Electrodiagnosis

Electroretinography (ERG)

The retina generates a potential which can be measured using a gold foil electrode in contact with the cornea over the lower lid, or using a contact lens electrode. The potential is compared with a reference electrode, and the change in voltage produced by a light stimulus is called the electroretinogram (ERG). If the ambient illumination is photopic (bright), the response is largely generated by cones; cone response can be further selected by flicker stimulus at greater than 20 Hz. In scotopic (dim) illumination, the ERG is rod-driven. The ERG is a complex wave, in which two main components, the *a* and *b* waves, can be identified. The *a* wave principally reflects receptor function, while the *b* wave derives from the inner layers of the retina.

Electro-oculography (EOG)

The RPE generates a positive resting potential at the cornea relative to the periocular skin. This potential difference is greater in the light than in the dark, and in standardized conditions of adaptation the ratio between the light and dark potentials is called the Arden index (potential$_{light}$/potential$_{dark}$), and is a measure of RPE function. The Arden index is >185 per cent in normal subjects, and is reduced early in tapetoretinal degenerations.

EOG can also be used to record eye movements.

Visual evoked response (VER)

The VER (or potential) measures the velocity of conduction from the retina to the occipital cortex (as latency), and the amplitude of the cortical response. Pattern stimulus evokes a greater response than flash, and both are generally used in clinical VER testing. Latency measures optic nerve conduction velocity, and is normally <120 ms; it is increased in demyelinating optic nerve disease. Amplitude is a more variable quantity, because it is influenced by the testing procedure. It is reduced in cortical disease, and may be asymmetric in lateralized occipital cortical infarct causing hemianopia.

Recommended further reading

Chopdar, A. (1989). *Manual of fundus fluorescein angiography*. Butterworths, London.

Desmedt, J.E. (ed.) (1990). Visual evoked potentials. *Clinical neurophysiology updates* Vol. 3. Elsevier, Amsterdam.

Duane, T.D. (1976). *Clinical ophthalmology*. Harper & Row, Philadelphia. Revised annually.

Fraunfelder and Roy. (1990). *Current ocular therapy* 3. W.B. Saunders, Philadelphia.

Gonzalez, C.F., Becker, M.M., and Flanagan, J.C. (ed.) (1986). *Diagnostic imaging in ophthalmology*. Springer Verlag, New York.

Guthoff, R. (1991). *Ultrasound in ophthalmological diagnosis. A practical guide*. Thieme Verlag, New York.

Huber, M.J.E. and Reacher, M.H. (1990). *Clinical tests. Ophthalmology*. Wolfe, London.

Kanski, J.J. (1988). *Clinical ophthalmology*, 2nd edn. Butterworths, London.

Miller, S. (1987). *Clinical ophthalmology*. Wright, Bristol.

Reese, A. (1976). *Tumours of the eye*. Harper & Row, Hagerstown.

Spalton, D.J., Hitchings, R.A., and Hunter, P.A. (1985). *Atlas of clinical ophthalmology*. Churchill Livingstone, Edinburgh.

Weale, R.A. (1982). *A biography of the eye*. Lewis, London.

2
Eyelids and external diseases

The eyelids

Anatomy

The eyelids form the anterior boundary of the orbit (divided by a horizontal aperture, the palpebral fissure). The orbital septum joins the tarsal plate of each lid to the periosteum of the orbital margin, with which it is continuous; thickenings of this fibrous layer form the medial and lateral canthal ligaments, which sling the lids from their bony attachments on the medial and lateral orbital walls. The medial ligament divides to surround the upper part of the lacrimal sac and insert into the anterior and posterior lacrimal crests. The tarsal plates form the 'skeleton' of the eyelids, and the orbital septum separates the tissues of the orbit from superficial preseptal tissues.

Orbicularis lies anterior to the tarsal plate and septum (as the pretarsal and preseptal orbicularis, respectively); this muscle together with the vessels, subcutaneous tissues, and skin are collectively termed the anterior lamella. The posterior lamella comprises the tarsal plate and conjunctiva, with associated goblet cells, lash follicles, and Meibomian glands.

Levator palpebrae superioris (and its analogue in the lower lid) is inserted into the tarsal plate by an aponeurosis, and through the septum and orbicularis into the subcutaneous tissues to form the lid crease. Its origin is with that of superior rectus, at the orbital apex and it is innervated by the superior division of the III nerve. On its inferior surface is a thin, sympathetically innervated smooth muscle element (Müller's muscle), which contributes to the involuntary resting lid position.

Infection and inflammation

Blepharitis

The lids may be involved in allergic, infective, or seborrhoeic inflammation.

Allergic blepharitis is common in atopic patients, causing acute lid swelling together with allergic conjunctivitis. Allergic contact dermatitis involving the eyelids commonly follows topical therapy, and may be due to the active pharmacological agent (especially atropine and neomycin), or to the preservatives (e.g. benzalkonium) used in the preparation.

Blepharitis is often associated with infection by *Staphylococcus aureus* or *epidermidis*, although it may not be clear whether the infection is the primary cause of the blepharitis or a secondary superinfection. Associated marginal corneal ulcers suggest staphylococcal involvement, and are caused by hyper-sensitivity to bacterial toxin. These eyes require treatment with antibiotic (chlor-amphenicol topically or flucloxacillin orally) and topical steroid.

Viral causes of blepharitis include herpes simplex (vesiculation of eyelid skin, especially in children, as a primary herpes infection), and herpes zoster (vesiculation and crusting in a dermatomal distribution). Molluscum contagiosum is a white umbilicated lid margin mass caused by viral infection of the basal layer of lid epidermis; it is sometimes associated with follicular conjunctivitis, pannus or corneal epitheliopathy.

Non-infective, non-allergic blepharitis occurs in seborrhoeic individuals, in whom an accumulation of sebum and squames clings to the lashes and lid margins, sometimes with secondary bacterial infection. Frequent lid scrubs using neutral shampoo on a cotton wool bud eliminate the accumulations, but secondary infection may require antibiotic treatment.

Rosacea involves the lids in a more general facial vascular hyper-reactivity, with telangiectasia, acneiform dermatitis, and sensitivity to triggers such as coffee. There is often associated corneal epitheliopathy, and the condition usually responds well to treatment with oral tetracycline over several weeks.

Stye

Infection (usually staphylococcal) of the gland of Zeis, or a lash follicle, causing localized acute inflammation on the external surface of the lid, sometimes with abscess formation. Treat styes by epilation of the involved lash and antibiotic ointment. A large abscess may require incision and drainage as well as antibiotic.

Chalazion (Meibomian cyst)

Localized lid swelling, containing accumulated tarsal gland secretions. Chalazia are palpable, and seen on the tarsal (inner) surface of the lid (cf. styes), but they are also visible externally, and sometimes cause cosmetic complaint. They usually resolve spontaneously but often recur, and are treated definitively by incision (vertically, through tarsal surface of lid), and curettage.

Sebaceous cyst

Sebaceous cysts on the eyelids are common, and are removed under local anaesthesia.

Lid margin malposition

Contact between the lid margin and the surface of the eye ensures a stable and evenly spread tear film which is regularly replaced during blinking, and also that the tears drain into the lacrimal sac by maintaining apposition between the puncta and the lacus of tears. Correct lid margin position is maintained by a balance between everting (levator) and inverting (orbicularis) forces. This balance may be disturbed by atrophic (involutional) or cicatrizing changes.

Lower lid margin malposition is most commonly due to involutional weakening of the lid muscles, or change in the anatomical relationship of orbicularis to the tarsal plate. Correction is achieved by surgical restoration of the balance, by strengthening of retractors' everting action (in entropion), or shortening the lid margin and removing excess laxity in orbicularis (in ectropion).

In the upper lid, weakness of levator or involutional dehiscence of its aponeurosis causes ptosis.

Conjunctival cicatrization

Conjunctival scarring and contraction beneath the tarsal plate may follow chronic inflammation (pemphigoid, erythema multiforme, trachoma, chemical burns). If this occurs beneath the upper lid (which occurs typically in trachoma), upper lid entropion follows, and leads to trichiasis and corneal ulceration and scarring. Cicatrization involving the lid skin (burn, tumour, irradiation), increases the everting force on the lid, leading to ectropion.

Entropion

Aetiology

Senile (spastic) entropion affects the lower lids, and is caused by laxity of the retractor and its aponeurosis, allowing unopposed orbicularis to ride over the lid margin, rolling it into inversion.

Cicatricial entropion follows scarring secondary to chemical burn, pemphigoid, or repeated surgical trauma, especially repeated attempts at cryoablation of lashes.

Treatment

Wies procedure (full-thickness horizontal section of the lid through the upper one third of the tarsal plate, and plication of the retractor through the tarsotomy to the anterior surface of the tarsal plate and skin) is most often successful in effecting permanent cure of senile entropion. Numerous other surgical procedures are described. Temporary relief may be achieved by taping down the lid with light adhesive tape. Cicatricial entropion often requires more elaborate oculoplastic surgery.

Rotation of the tarsal margin through 90° is an elegant solution to most minor degrees of upper lid entropion, but if cicatrization is severe, mucous membrane autograft, may be necessary.

Ectropion

Abnormal lower lid eversion, causing accumulation of tears, failure of drainage, and epiphora (watering eye), which is often complicated by secondary infection. Ectropion is caused by flaccid involution of orbicularis, often associated with functional excess lid margin length, or skin cicatrization.

Treatment

Surgical correction is indicated if the ectropion produces symptoms. The aim of surgery is to reduce the length of the lid margin and take up laxity in orbicularis.

This is achieved in the modified Kuhnt–Zymanowski procedure by full thickness base-up wedge resection combined with reinsertion temporally of the freed skin flap, or by plication of the medial or lateral canthal ligaments to periosteum. Ectropion limited to the medial part of the lower lid produces punctal eversion and epiphora; it is corrected surgically by retropunctal cautery or diamond-shaped excision of tarsus below the punctum, avoiding the inferior canaliculus.

Trichiasis

Eyelashes touch and abrade the cornea if they grow inwards. This may occur:

(1) in association with entropion;
(2) as aberrant lashes (isolated);
(3) in distichiasis (if they form a more or less complete secondary lash line).

They irritate, cause surface irritation, watering (epiphora), superficial punctate keratopathy (SPK), epithelial ulceration, corneal neovascularization, ulceration, and scarring.

Trichiasis secondary to entropion is managed by correction of the entropion.

Epilation (removal of lashes with forceps) is usually effective only for one or two isolated aberrant lashes. The trichiasis usually recurs, and the regrowing lash stumps are often increasingly troublesome. Electrolysis is very effective if adequate. Successful electrolysis requires good local anaesthesia, and sufficient power completely to destroy the follicles. The electrolysis probe is introduced 1–2 mm into the follicle adjacent to the lash, and the current turned on for 3–8 s to produce coagulation (indicated by bubbling at the lash base). The successfully treated lash can be removed without resistance. Recurrence after a few weeks indicates inadequate treatment.

Cryotherapy is sometimes used when electrolysis has failed. Two or three cycles of freeze–thaw are produced with a special broad, low temperature probe applied to the lid margin. Follicles are destroyed at −20°C, while basal cells and blood vessels are spared. Repeated applications of cryo may lead to scarring and cicatricial entropion.

Ptosis

Ptosis may be congenital or acquired, unilateral or bilateral, and give rise to visual or cosmetic symptoms.

Aetiology

Congenital

- levator weakness,
- congenital Horner's syndrome.

Acquired

- involutional   weakness, dehiscence or disinsertion of the aponeurosis from levator and the tarsal plate

- neurogenic   III nerve palsy (partial or complete)
              Horner's syndrome
              myasthenia
- myogenic   ocular myopathy
- mechanical tumours, masses and inflammation of the upper lid
- traumatic   disinsertion of levator aponeurosis.

Pseudoptosis

- enophthalmos,
- microphthalmos,
- phthisis,
- hypertropia or contralateral hypotropia,
- lacrimal gland tumour,
- Duane's lid-retraction syndrome,
- contralateral proptosis or pseudoproptosis,
- eyelid inflammation.

Assessment

1. Measure the degree of ptosis and levator function. Use a ruler while eliminating frontalis contribution to lid excursion by firm pressure on the brow.
2. Check external ocular movements and pupils, for III palsy and Horner's syndrome.
3. Test corneal sensation and Bell's phenomenon.
4. Exclude complex ocular motility disorder (Marcus–Gunn jaw-winking; Duane's lid-retraction syndrome) and myasthenia.

Degree of ptosis (Fig. 2.1)

The difference between the heights of each lid in the primary position. If the ptosis is bilateral, assume that the normal position of the upper lid margin is 2 mm below the limbus at 12 o'clock.

- mild ptosis   less than 2 mm,
- moderate ptosis 2–4 mm,
- severe ptosis   more than 4 mm.

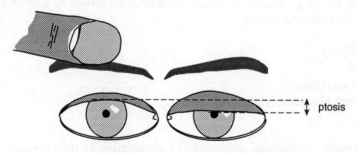

Fig. 2.1   Measurement of ptosis.

Levator function (Fig. 2.2)

Levator function is measured as lid excursion, i.e. the difference in height of the upper lid margin between maximum up- and down-gaze.

- good   more than 8 mm,
- fair   5–8 mm,
- poor   less than 5 mm.

Management

Indications for surgery

Functional

Obstruction of visual axis. Children with ptosis may be at risk of stimulus-deprivation amblyopia.

Cosmetic

Generally, the less severe the defect, the more likely a patient will find the result of a plastic procedure undertaken for cosmetic reasons unsatisfactory.

Surgical principles

Congenital ptosis

Lid surgery in children must be performed under general anaesthesia. Over-correction is not usually a problem, and the procedure is planned according to the degree of ptosis and levator function (Table 2.1).

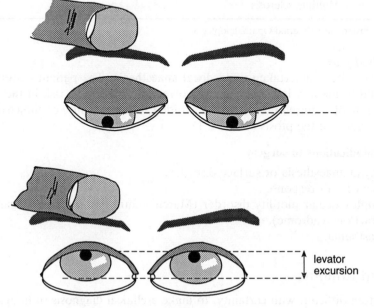

levator
excursion

Fig. 2.2   Measurement of levator excursion.

Table 2.1 Surgical correction of ptosis

	Ptosis	Levator function	Procedure
Congenital	mild	always good	no surgery Fasanella small (10–12 mm) levator resection
	moderate	good fair	14–17 mm levator resection 18–20 mm levator resection
	severe	fair poor	20 mm levator resection frontalis sling
Acquired	Horner's syndrome		Fasanella
	senile		Fasanella levator resection 8–10 mm if moderate ptosis and moderate to good levator function.
	PEO		no surgery—absent Bell's phenomenon ptosis crutch
	Myasthenia		no surgery
	After cataract surgery		Fasanella

	Traumatic
	  early
	  late
			
			levator reinsertion
			brow suspension

	Multiple sclerosis		no surgery

PEO = Progressive External Ophthalmoplegia

Acquired ptosis
Surgery is best undertaken under local anaesthesia. The patient's cooperation is useful to identify levator, and overcorrection, which is a risk in the surgical correction of acquired ptosis, can be avoided. The procedure of choice depends on the cause of the ptosis (Table 2.1).

Contraindications to surgery
- corneal anaesthesia or surface disorder,
- absent Bell's response,
- complex ocular motility disorder (Marcus–Gunn jaw-winking, Duane's lid-retraction syndrome),
- myasthenia.

Eyelid tumours

It is often difficult, with certainty, to make a clinical diagnosis of lumps on the eyelids. If there is any doubt they should be excised or biopsied. If basal or squamous cell carcinoma or melanoma is a possibility, excision should include a margin of clinically healthy tissue; clinical recurrence is not uncommon in spite of this margin. All excised tissue should be sent, whole, for histology.

Benign tumours

Keratoacanthoma (KA)

Benign hyperplasia of the epidermis with exuberant keratin production. The clinical appearance of KA is variable, but the edges are generally well demarcated. KA may grow alarmingly rapidly and become very large. Treat by biopsy and curettage or excision.

Molluscum contagiosum

Single or multiple nodules with central umbilication, caused by virally induced inflammation and proliferation of epidermal cells. Conjunctivitis or keratitis associated with mollusca on the lid margin resolves with excision of the molluscum.

Malignant tumours

Basal cell carcinoma (BCC)

Pleomorphic, locally invasive tumours. BCC classically presents with raised, rolled edges and a pearly centre, but may be extensive and non-ulcerating, with a diffuse area of indurated, fibrotic, discoloured skin (morphoeic), or is occasionally cystic. Exposure to sunlight may contribute in the aetiology of some cases of BCC. Treat by wide surgical excision (confirm complete removal by histology of the edges of the lesion) and clinical follow-up to monitor for recurrence. Alternative approaches to treatment include temperature-monitored nitrogen cryotherapy or radiotherapy. These modalities may be especially useful if a large section of lid margin, or the canaliculi, are involved. Radiotherapy is unsuitable for upper lid tumours since it may be followed by conjunctival keratinization, and secondary keratopathy. Plastic surgical lid reconstruction may be necessary following excision of a large tumour.

Untreated BCC invades adjacent tissues relentlessly. Occasionally, BCC is multifocal and recurrent (BCC—naevus syndrome). Treatment of periocular tumours should then be co-ordinated with plastic surgery and radiotherapy.

Squamous cell carcinoma (SCC)

SCC is a less common lid tumour than BCC, and presents with a very variable clinical appearance, often resembling non-specific chronic inflammation, with or without ulceration, which may be multifocal. Blood-borne metastasis occurs if the tumour penetrates the basement membrane to involve the dermis. Treatment is by wide surgical excision.

Melanoma

The natural history of lid melanoma depends on the depth of involvement and the degree of cellular anaplasia. There is a continuous spectrum from the nonmitotic, static naevus, which is entirely intra-epidermal, through junctional naevi involving the deepest layer of the epidermis and breaking through the basement membrane into the dermis, to frankly malignant tumours. Pigmentation is variable, and not a useful prognostic sign.

Change in thickness or size indicates mitotic activity, and these tumours should be excised.

Exposure to solar radiation is implicated as an aetiological factor in BCC and SCC, and in melanoma.

Tear film disorders and dry eye

Physiology

The tears cover the cornea to give an optically perfect anterior refracting surface, and prevent desiccation and corneal epithelial damage. SPK, ulceration and perforation can occur quickly if corneal surface wetting is compromised; corneas of patients with rheumatoid disease are at particular risk of perforation.

The tear film is maintained by blinking, and after circulating over the surface of the eye it forms a meniscus at the lower lid margin. This drains via the puncta into the canaliculi and the lacrimal sac. Normally the lower canaliculus drains up to 80 per cent of the tears, but a normal upper canaliculus can often drain all the tears if the lower system is obstructed. The sac drains via the nasolacrimal duct into the nasopharynx, beneath the inferior turbinate. In addition, a variable proportion of the tear film is lost by evaporation, and epiphora (watering) is especially troublesome when evaporation is reduced or tear flow is increased (e.g. in cold, windy weather). Lid margin malposition (entropion or ectropion), or obstruction of the lacrimal drainage system, interfere with normal tear drainage.

The tear film has three component layers:

1. *Mucous*, secreted by conjunctival goblet cells. Mucin wets the brush border of the corneal epithelial cells, making their surface hydrophilic and stabilizing the tear film. Mucin deficiency (linear IgA disease, xerophthalmia) prevents epithelial wetting and allows rapid tear film breakup.
2. *Aqueous*, the thickest component, secreted by the lacrimal glands. The aqueous phase of the tear film carries immune cells and IgA, and is deficient in rheumatoid, Sjögren's, sarcoid, neoplastic lacrimal gland infiltration (Miculicz), and Parinaud's oculoglandular syndrome.
3. *Lipid*, the surface layer derived from Meibomian secretion, which retards tear film evaporation.

Dry eye

Deficiency of any of the three components of the tear film causes functional wetting inadequacy, and leads to symptoms and signs of dry eye. Dry eyes are common in the elderly, reflecting a reduction in all three components or a disturbance in the balance between them. There may be a paradoxical lacrimal hypersecretion in response to tear film instability, or mucus overproduction in the face of lacrimal hyposecretion.

Symptoms

Itching, burning, grittiness, foreign body sensation.

Signs

Staining

Rose Bengal stains dead and diseased epithelial cells, and mucin, and is a more sensitive indicator in the assessment of dry eye than fluorescein. Punctate staining of the inferior cornea and conjunctiva indicate functional tear film deficiency. Excess tear film debris (mucus and epithelial debris) is an important indication of dry eye.

Tear film breakup

The normal tear film is stable for more than 15 s if blinking is voluntarily suspended; breakup in less than 10 s indicates instability which will cause dry eye symptoms, and may lead to epithelial drying and focal ulceration. Breakup time is measured by staining the tear film with fluorescein, and timing the appearance of the first break in the stained tear film illuminated with blue light at the slit-lamp. It is a sign of reduced mucus function, or surface keratinization.

Schirmer's test

This measures lacrimal secretion by the amount of its absorption (measured in millimetres) on a strip of filter paper in 5 min. Less than 5 mm wetting is considered to indicate impaired lacrimal gland function. Schirmer's test demonstrates gross reduction in the aqueous component of the tear film but is not very accurate, and cannot detect functional tear film problems in which lacrimal secretion is not reduced.

Management

Most dry eyes have no identifiable cause, but underlying rheumatoid or other connective tissue disorder must be managed appropriately if present. The aim of treatment is symptomatic relief and protection of the corneal epithelium. Many artificial tear substitutes are available; none has clear advantages over the others, though patients often have preferences. It is reasonable to begin with hypromellose, and try others if this fails to give relief. Artificial tears should be used freely, as often as necessary, and the most common reason for their failure is inadequate use. Lubricating ointment (oc. simplex) can be used for longer effect at night. Artificial tears containing acetylcysteine, which has a mucolytic effect, are useful to remove mucus accumulation, in filamentary keratitis and in ulcer craters.

Watering eye (epiphora)

Caused by tear production in excess of drainage capacity.

Aetiology

Overproduction

Reflex lacrimation caused by surface irritation. Any anatomical, mechanical, traumatic, or inflammatory disorder of cornea, conjunctiva, or lid may stimulate increased tear production. Epiphora is then a symptom of the underlying condition.

Under-drainage

Malposition of the punctum, caused by ectropion affecting either the entire lower lid, or only its medial part.

Occlusion in the lacrimal drainage system can occur at the punctum, lower, upper, or common canaliculus, lacrimal sac or nasolacrimal duct (NLD). It is most commonly due to outflow obstruction at the NLD in association with chronic inflammation in the sinuses or nasopharynx, but may also be congenital (delayed canalization of the NLD), traumatic or inflammatory, or occasionally due to tumour. Intermittent symptoms, often present only in cold or windy weather, are due to functional obstruction (reduced drainage facility which is able to cope with normal tear production), and are often not sufficiently troublesome to warrant surgery. Swelling over the lacrimal sac in association with a watering eye may be due to mucocoele, infection, or tumour. Firm pressure over a mucocoele causes mucus regurgitation through one or both puncta. Dacryocystitis presents with acute inflammation over the sac and purulent discharge; this may become recurrent or chronic, leading to drainage obstruction, mucocoele formation, and chronic epiphora. Malignancy (adenocarcinoma, SCC, or lymphoma) should be suspected in chronic drainage obstruction associated with a mass over the sac, especially if it extends above the medial canthal ligament, or if the tears are blood-stained.

Assessment

1. How serious are the symptoms?
2. Is there a non-obstructive cause?
3. If not, where is the obstruction?
4. Is there associated dacryocystitis or mucocoele?

Tear duct syringing

Under topical anaesthesia, dilate the lower punctum with a Nettleship's dilator passed downward for 1 mm, and then medially for 2–3 mm. Pull the outer canthus laterally to tension the lid margin (preventing kinking of the canaliculus), pass a lacrimal cannula on a syringe into the canaliculus until its tip gently meets resistance at the medial wall of the sac, and irrigate gently with sterile saline. If fluid passes into the nasopharynx the system is anatomically patent. Regurgitation through the upper canaliculus indicates obstruction at the nasolacrimal duct, sac, or common canaliculus.

Management

Lid malposition

- trichiasis   electrolysis, cryotherapy, tarsal margin rotation,
- entropion   Wies procedure,
- flaccid ectropion   Kuhnt–Szymanowski operation,
- cicatricial ectropion   oculoplastic procedures, e.g. Z-plasty,
- medial ectropion   retropunctal cautery or wedge resection.

Punctal stenosis

Dilatation, three-snip procedure.

Obstruction

Dacryocystorhinostomy (DCR)
DCR provides definitive surgical cure in appropriate cases. The operation is only indicated if epiphora causes significant symptoms, and is best avoided in elderly patients.

NLD obstruction is often associated with rhinitis and sinusitis, and sinus X-rays and an ENT opinion may be useful before undertaking DCR. Intubation of the DCR with an O'Donoghue's tube (actually a solid silastic splint) maintains patency of the anastamosis between sac and nasopharynx during healing; the tube is left *in situ* for 6 months, unless previously expelled. The tubes may partially prolapse, presenting with a redundant loop in the medial canthus. This can seldom be reduced by pushing the tubes back through the canaliculi from above, but they can sometimes be located beneath the middle turbinate by an ENT surgeon, and pulled back into place. If this is impossible they must be divided in the medial canthus and trimmed, and will ultimately be passed through the nose. Some surgeons use a tube only if there is canalicular obstruction or stenosis.

Dacryocystitis and mucocoele

Treat the infection acutely with a broad spectrum antibiotic with anti-staphylococcal activity (e.g. ampicillin and flucloxacillin), beginning with intravenous treatment if the infection is severe. Plan DCR (or in the elderly sometimes dacryocystectomy) when the acute inflammation is controlled. It may be necessary to drain the sac in acute dacryocystitis.

Occasionally chronic dacryocystitis is associated with actinomycotic infection, and yellow 'sulphur granules' are found in the sac at DCR. Though actinomyces is sensitive to pencillin, surgical drainage is sufficient to clear the infection, and specific antimicrobial therapy is not necessary.

Lacrimal sac tumours

Tumours may be unsuspected, and discovered only during surgery. Treatment is by complete dacryocystectomy, followed by radiotherapy.

Conjunctiva

The conjunctiva is a mucous membrane covering the anterior sclera (bulbar conjunctiva), and is reflected in the fornices to cover the tarsal surfaces of the lids (tarsal conjunctiva). Its epithelial layer is continuous with the corneal epithelium, and the bulbar conjunctiva is intimately related to Tenon's capsule for 2–3 mm around the limbus.

Conjunctivitis

The tarsal conjunctiva contains goblet cells within the mucosa (epithelium), and lymphoid tissue in the submucosa. Inflammation gives rise to a papillary or follicular reaction.

Papillae consist of hyperplastic epithelium with a central capillary frond. They are a reaction to infection, allergy, trauma, chemical or contact lens-associated irritation, and do not provide an aetiological diagnosis. Follicles are submucosal foci of lymphatic proliferation, which are avascular, and are seen particularly in viral, chlamydial, and chronic allergic conditions.

Bullous and membranous conjunctivitis occasionally occur in immunologically based inflammation (Stevens–Johnson syndrome, pemphigoid, ligneous conjunctivitis).

Acute conjunctivitis

Ask for history of allergy and exposure to irritants, and exclude other causes of acute red eye, particularly keratitis and anterior uveitis, by slit-lamp examination. Examine exudate in inferior fornix, and swab for culture, if indicated, before using fluorescein, local anaesthetic, or antibiotic.

Symptoms

Red eye, gritty discomfort, associated with serous, mucoid, or purulent discharge, stickiest on waking. Vision is unaffected and there is no photophobia, unless there is coexisting keratitis. Generalized influenza-like symptoms often occur in viral conjunctivitis.

Signs

Engorgement of surface vessels over entire conjunctiva, including tarsal surfaces of lids, and chemosis (conjunctival oedema). Evert the upper lid to show papillary or follicular reaction. Viral conjunctivitis may be associated with pre-auricular lymphadenopathy (adenovirus), conjunctival haemorrhage (Cocksackievirus and enterovirus), and follicular subtarsal reaction. Pannus (neovascularization of the upper limbus) is a feature of chlamydial conjunctivitis, and also occurs in wearers of soft contact lenses.

Investigation

Swab for culture and Gram stain if the infection is unresponsive to treatment, associated with corneal pathology, or follows intraocular surgery. If chlamydia is suspected, scrape lesions from the tarsal surface of the everted upper lid with the edge of a scalpel blade, transferring half into culture medium and the remainder on to a microscope slide. Serological examination for chlamydia antigen, or microscopic identification of inclusion bodies in epithelial cells, confirms chlamydial aetiology.

Treatment

Bacterial

Treat with a broad spectrum topical antibiotic (chloramphenicol, soframycin) unless more specific therapy is mandated by clinical failure to respond and culture. Drops need to be used frequently (2-hourly) initially to maintain effective tissue levels and produce a satisfactory response. Therapeutic levels are maintained by less frequent (4–6 hourly) application of ointment, although the smearing it produces may not be tolerable by day. Antibiotics such as gentamicin, which have important systemic use, are best avoided as first-line broad spectrum treatment, to avoid selection of resistant bacteria.

Chlamydia

Chlamydia is the commonest cause of ophthalmia neonatorum, and is sexually acquired in adults. Extraocular infection occurs in both neonatal and adult chlamydial conjunctivitis, and topical tetracycline (oc. tetracycline q.d.s. for 3 weeks) must be supplemented with systemic treatment (oral teracycline in adults, and oral erythromycin in infants) for 3 weeks. Adults with chlamydial infections should also be advised to have their sexual partners examined and treated, to avoid a cycle of reinfection.

Viral

Viral conjunctivitis is self-limiting, and no specific treatment is effective. Adenoviral keratoconjunctivitis takes weeks to resolve, during which symptomatic treatment with topical steroid may be helpful.

Allergic

Allergic conjunctivitis presents with rapidly increasing chemosis following exposure of an allergic individual to an allergen. Topical steroids reduce the inflammation, and sodium cromoglycate inhibits the inflammatory response to exogenous allergens. Begin treatment with steroid, adding cromoglycate when the inflammation is controlled, and reducing the strength and frequency of steroid according to clinical response. Use steroid without combined antibiotic to minimize antigenic challenge to inflamed atopic tissues.

Chronic conjunctivitis

Vernal conjunctivitis

Vernal conjunctivitis is a chronic follicular inflammation in atopic individuals, usually with no specific relation to an identifiable allergen. Children are usually most severely affected, the inflammation reducing gradually into adulthood. Symptoms are variable, and may decrease if potential sources of allergen (e.g. furry pets) are removed.

The tarsal surface of the upper lids is irregular, with follicles and epithelial inflammation, and mucous plaques accumulate on the cornea. These surface irregularities cause gritty discomfort and may reduce vision considerably, also causing ptosis and photophobia. Treat with topical steroid (dexamethasone) initially, monitoring the effectiveness of treatment by observing the response of the follicles. As the condition is chronic, and prolonged topical steroid carries significant risk of complication, reduce the frequency of this treatment as soon as possible once the symptoms are controlled.

Contact lens-associated conjunctivitis

Contact lens wear constitutes a chronic irritative stimulus to the surface of the eye. In addition soft contact lenses often contain residues of their cleaning and storage fluids, and protein residues derived from the tear film.

Surface anoxia is a common acute problem in hard lens wearers, reduced by the higher water content (and therefore greater permeability) of gas-permeable lenses. It presents with punctate corneal epitheliopathy, and resolves within days to a period of discontinuation of lens wear.

Giant papillary conjunctivitis is exclusively a contact lens-associated disorder, which presents with large subtarsal papillae (foci of vascular epithelial hypertrophy). There is often associated pannus (superior limbal neovascularization). Lens wear must be discontinued for months, or permanently.

Cicatrizing conjunctivitis

Mucous membrane pemphigoid and the Stevens–Johnson syndrome cause bullous conjunctival ulceration, followed by progressive submucosal fibrosis, leading to cicatrization and symblepharon. Ultimately much of the normal conjunctiva is lost, together with its goblet cells, leading to lid deformity, dry eye and exposure keratopathy, and secondarily to corneal scarring and opacification.

Conjunctival bullae in pemphigoid are caused by breakdown of the desmosomes, which attach the basal layer of mucosal cells to the conjunctival basement membrane. IgA and IgM are deposited on the basement membrane in a type II hypersensitivity reaction, with activation of complement, leading to submucosal infiltration, progressive fibrosis and scarring, cicatrization and symblepharon.

Stevens–Johnson syndrome disease is a type III hypersensitivity (circulating antigen–antibody complex) vasculitis, which can be stimulated by a variety of antigens, including drugs (notably sulphonamides), viruses, and bacteria. It begins as a general febrile illness, followed by a skin rash and bullous eruption affecting all mucous membranes, particularly the mouth and conjunctiva.

Treatment of neither condition is entirely satisfactory. In the acute phase, intensive topical steroids help stabilize the mucosa, and antibiotic ointment is given to prevent secondary bacterial infection. In the longer term, artificial tears protect against the effects of the secondary tear film disorder, and lid surgery may be necessary to correct cicatricial entropion.

Pigmented conjunctival lesions

Conjunctival naevus is common in pigmented races; melanoma is uncommon. Signs of malignancy in a pigmented conjunctival lesion are thickening, enlargement, and adjacent tissue distortion. Suspicious lesions should be biopsied or excised.

Adrenochrome pigmentation was a common sequela to long-term use of adrenalin drops in the treatment of glaucoma. Dipivefrin, which has largely replaced adrenalin in this context, does not lead to significant pigment production.

Pterygium

Pterygium is a fibrovascular proliferation extending horizontally across the cornea from the nasal conjunctiva. Its removal is indicated on cosmetic grounds, or if it threatens the visual axis; outside the tropics this is rare. It is more commonly of cosmetic concern, and reassurance that it is benign and not a threat is often all that is needed. It is removed surgically by excising the entire corneal part of the lesion (down to Bowman's membrane), as well as all abnormal conjunctiva. Recurrence is common.

Disorders involving periocular skin

Rosacea

Rosacea is a condition in which multiple facial telangiectasia, especially around the eyes and nose are associated with facial flushing in response to xanthines (e.g. in coffee). In extreme cases there is hypertrophy of the soft tissue of the nose (rhinophyma). Rosacea is associated with chronic superficial keratitis, leading to vascularization and scarring, especially of the inferior half of the cornea. Tetracycline in low dose over a long period, and topical steroids, may reduce the inflammation and suppress neovascularization.

Herpes zoster ophthalmicus

This presents with erythema distributed over the V_1 dermatome, associated with and often preceded by pain. It is usually unilateral, respecting the midline, but may be bilateral. Vesicular ulceration and skin inflammation may be severe, and the ulcerative phase may last for weeks or months. Involvement of the tip of the nose indicates nasociliary nerve involvement, and an increased risk of anterior uveitis.

Oral and topical acyclovir are reported to reduce the severity of the attack if given very early in its course (usually earlier than ophthalmic presentation), but have no effect on postherpetic neuralgia.

Ocular zoster

Cornea

Herpes zoster causes reduced corneal sensation and microdendritic ulceration, but unlike herpes simplex does not lead to corneal destruction. Topical acyclovir may hasten healing of zoster epitheliopathy. Neurotrophic keratitis may be a late problem.

Anterior uveitis

Treatment of zoster uveitis can be a delicate management problem. It may be severe, and characteristically leads to posterior synaechia formation, iris atrophy, cataract and secondary glaucoma. Mydriatics give symptomatic relief and reduce the risk of synaechia causing pupil block. Topical steroids are necessary if the inflammation is vigorous, but their withdrawal may be difficult and must be gradual. Some patients require maintenance with low level steroid treatment (as little as 0.01 per cent predsol twice a week for months) to prevent recurrence. On this account topical steroids should not be commenced in patients with zoster except to treat uveitis.

Zoster neuropathy

Paresis of any of the extraocular motor nerves may complicate zoster and produce diplopia. Zoster infection of the geniculate ganglion involves the facial nerve as it passes through the internal auditory meatus, producing the Ramsay Hunt syndrome (ipsilateral facial weakness, reduced tear production, and hyperacusis).

Prolonged pain in the distribution of the affected sensory division is characteristic of zoster and may be difficult to treat. Analgesics may be supplemented with carbamazepine or tricyclics, and in severe cases the collaboration of the pain clinic may be helpful.

Recommended further reading

Beard, C. (1981). Ptosis, 3rd edn. Mosby, St Louis.
Chandler, J.W., Sugar, J., and Edelhauser, H.F. (1994). External diseases: cornea, conjunctiva, sclera, eyelids, lacrimal system. (Vol. 8, Textbook of ophthalmology (ed. S.M. Podos and M. Yanoff.) Mosby, St Louis.
Donaldson (1980). Atlas of external diseases of the eye, Vol. III, 2nd edn, Cornea & sclera. Mosby, St Louis.
Dutton (1989). A colour atlas of ptosis. PG Publishing, Singapore.

Easty, D.L. and Smolin, G. (1985). *External eye diseases*. Butterworths, London.
Ostler, H.B. (1993). *Diseases of the external eye and adnexa. A text and atlas*. Williams and Wilkins, Baltimore.
Polack, F.M. (1991). *External diseases of the eye*. Scriba, Barcelona.
Tabbara, K.F. and Hyndvik, R.A. (1986). *Infection of the eye*. Little, Brown & Co., Boston.
Watts, M.T. and Nelson, M.E. (1992). *External eye disease: a colour atlas*. Churchill Livingstone, Edinburgh.

3

The anterior segment

Cornea

Anatomy and physiology

Epithelium

The corneal epithelium is a stratified non-keratinized epithelium, some six cells thick. Young cells migrate towards the centre from stem cells at the limbus. During centripetal migration they proliferate and mature, from deep to superficial, to replace those lost by desquamation or trauma. Adjacent cells are joined by tight junctions, and basal cells are attached to the basement membrane by hemidesmosomes. Langerhans cells in the corneal epithelium express MHC antigens which may be important in graft rejection.

The corneal surface is covered by the tear film, which is 7 μm thick and has three layers:

1. A hydrophilic inner mucous layer which is produced by conjunctival goblet cells. It 'wets' the surface of the epithelial cell microvilli.
2. A middle aqueous layer produced by the lacrimal glands, containing immunoglobulins and enzymes, as well as white cells during inflammation.
3. An outer lipid layer, produced by the Meibomian glands in the eyelids, which reduces the rate of evaporation of the tear film and gives it surface stability.

Stroma

The stroma comprises 90 per cent of the total corneal thickness. It consists of an ordered arrangement of type I collagen fibres within a matrix of the glycosaminoglycans, keratan and chondroitin sulphate, and cells (keratocytes, Schwann cells). It is condensed to form Bowman's membrane at its outer border, to which the basement membrane (type IV collagen) of the epithelium is applied. Bowman's membrane separates epithelium from stroma, and is visible at the slit-lamp. Nerve fibres occur in the anterior and middle thirds of stroma. On its deep surface the stroma is separated by Descemet's membrane from the endothelium.

Endothelium

The endothelium is a single layer of hexagonal cells which are joined by discontinuous tight junctions, and are therefore permeable to some molecules, and water. The endothelial cells form a continuous sheet and are non-regenerating under physiological conditions. If their numbers are depleted (by surgery, trauma, or dystrophy), the remaining endothelial cells enlarge to fill the defect. Optical transparency is determined by the state of relative dehydration of the stroma, and depends on the balance between hydrating and dehydrating forces (see below).

Fluid transport across the cornea

Aqueous enters the stroma under hydrostatic aqueous pressure (IOP) and the colloid osmotic pressure gradient between aqueous and corneal stroma. At physiological steady state these factors are related by the equation:

$$IP = IOP - SP$$

where
IP   = imbibition pressure (the suction exerted by cannulated corneal stroma on extracorneal saline)
IOP = intraocular pressure
SP   = swelling pressure (the pressure which must be applied to prevent stromal swelling by increasing hydration).

Fluid is pumped from the stroma into the anterior chamber by the endothelium, and a small amount is lost to the exterior by evaporation. Corneal overhydration, leading to corneal oedema, is caused by functional or quantitative reduction in endothelial cell function below a critical level, or increase in IOP. Aqueous flow into the stroma then exceeds the endothelium's dehydrating capacity, and decompensation results.

Clinical presentation of corneal disease

Symptoms

Pain, photophobia (due to secondary anterior uveitis) and lacrimation are caused by trauma and acute inflammation.

Visual impairment—particularly dazzling by direct light—occurs when the optical clarity of the cornea is reduced. This can be caused by chronic (metabolic diseases, some dystrophies, scarring) or acute (acute corneal decompensation and oedema) disorders.

Signs

General

Ciliary injection (engorged circumcorneal vessels)
May be focal or involve the entire corneal circumference and is a sign of keratitis or uveitis.

Corneal sensation

Test with a whiff of tissue or cotton wool while the patient looks up, before using topical anaesthetic. Test the affected before the normal eye, comparing the relative responses. Sensation is reduced in keratitis, especially caused by herpes virus or acanthamoeba, and in the presence of a trigeminal lesion.

Prolonged severe corneal anaesthesia leads to neurotrophic keratopathy.

Opacities

Shown by slit-lamp examination using focal and scleral scatter illumination. Note their depth (epithelial, stromal or endothelial), extent and density. Faint sub-epithelial opacities are best seen by retroillumination or scleral scatter.

Distinguish cellular infiltration (active inflammation) from lipid deposition (chronic neovascular leak) by high power biomicroscopy.

Epithelium

Staining

Vital dye staining highlights surface disorder.

1. *Fluorescein* is taken up by areas where interepithelial cell junctions are broken down, or stroma is exposed beneath an epithelial defect.
2. *Rose Bengal* is taken up by epithelial cells devitalized by virus infection or desiccation, and by mucus strands. It is a good indicator of dry eye.

Superficial punctate keratopathy (SPK) is shown by a fine stippled staining of the intact epithelium, indicating a region of surface cell disorder. It is a non-specific and reversible sign of surface irritation (inflammatory, infective, traumatic, chemical, dry eye).

Epithelial defects occur in ulcers, abrasions, and erosions. Note their shape, record their size (measure with the slit-lamp beam), and examine their edges. Inflammatory cell infiltrate beneath, or at the edges of, an epithelial defect indicates active stromal inflammation.

Cysts or bullae occur in corneal oedema, and may be focal or regional, or involve the entire corneal epithelium.

Stroma

Compare the stromal thickness of one cornea with that of the other.

Thickening

Thickening is caused by oedema, due to endothelial decompensation or inflammation. Stromal oedema is accompanied by epithelial oedema (bullous kerato-pathy).

Thinning

Corneal thinning occurs in:

- ulcers (with epithelial defect):   infective, chemical, inflammatory (Mooren's, rheumatoid, PAN),
- ectasia (intact epithelium):   keratoconus, Terrien's marginal degeneration,
- keratomalacia: nutritional (vitamin A deficiency/malnutrition/measles),
- dellen (intact epithelium, focal thinning due to stromal desiccation without tissue loss):   local tear film instability, often adjacent to a surface irregularity.

Neovascularization
New vessel formation is stimulated by inflammation, trauma, and soft contact lens wear. New vessels may be located deeply or superficially in the stroma. White lipid deposits may accumulate around neovascular fronds, as the lipid fraction of lipoprotein leaking from the vessels accumulates in the stroma.

Ghost (empty) vessels
Pale, empty vessels in deep stroma indicate long-resolved keratitis. They are characteristic of interstitial keratitis, but can be a feature of resolved chronic keratitis of any cause.

Cellular infiltration
Inflammatory cells migrate to foci of keratitis, indicating active inflammation (e.g. at an ulcer base). Clinical progress can be monitored by following the extent and density of infiltration.

Stromal opacities
Causes:

- scarring of inflammatory or traumatic foci (irregular and focal),
- metabolic deposits (diffuse, or associated with vascularized cornea),
- dystrophies (characteristic morphology, according to type, and by definition bilateral).

Endothelium

Keratic precipitates (KP)
Creamy white deposits scattered over the endothelial surface. They occur in uveitis, and represent aggregations of inflammatory cells. Their shape and distribution may indicate aetiology (see p. 115).

Pigment deposition
Release of iris pigment cells follows anterior segment surgery, trauma, and acute glaucoma, and occurs in the pigment dispersion syndrome.

Cornea guttata
Fine dark endothelial stippling, distinguished from pigment by high power biomicroscopy with specular illumination, which shows pitting of the endothelial surface. Guttata indicate reduced endothelial capacity, and may represent an early or subclinical form of Fuchs' endothelial dystrophy.

Superficial corneal disorders

The epithelium is exposed to the air, covered by the tear film, and in contact with the lids. Adverse conditions in any of these (mechanical, chemical and thermal, tear deficiency, infection, and inflammation) affect the epithelium.

Dry eye

A common ocular surface disorder, caused by an inadequate tear film. The defect may be due to:

(1) deficiency of any of the three tear components;
(2) lid disorder which prevents normal spreading, maintenance and renewal of the tear film;
(3) corneal epithelial abnormality.

Tear film disorders are further described in Chapter 2.

Corneal abrasion

A traumatic focal epithelial defect, giving rise to a clear-cut area of fluorescein staining without significant stromal cellular infiltration. Abrasions heal within 2 or 3 days unless secondarily infected. Treat epithelial abrasions with antibiotic ointment to lubricate the contact between lids and abraded cornea and prevent infection, and topical mydriatic to relieve discomfort caused by secondary pupil spasm.

Recurrent corneal erosion

A focal epithelial defect caused by defective adhesion of the basal layer of epithelial cells to their basement membrane, often following an abrasion, and commonly occurring in corneas with epithelial dystrophy. Symptoms, signs and treatment are the same as for abrasion. Discomfort typically begins and recurs on waking in the morning. Persistent recurrences may sometimes be stabilized by padding, bandage contact lens, or debridement.

Adenoviral keratoconjunctivitis

Follicular conjunctivitis featuring patchy subepithelial corneal cellular infiltrates, sometimes with focal conjunctival haemorrhages and anterior uveitis. Adenoviral keratitis presents with red, watering, gritty eyes, and photophobia, associated with a general febrile illness, preauricular lymphadenopathy and malaise.

No specific antiviral treatment is effective, but symptoms may be reduced by topical steroid treatment.

Thygeson's keratitis

Chronic coarse superficial punctate keratitis, the lesions being arranged in scattered clumps which stain with fluorescein. By contrast with adenoviral keratoconjunctivitis, Thygeson's causes few symptoms, and the disorder is principally epithelial. Aetiology is uncertain and the clinical course is chronic remitting and relapsing. Topical steroids give symptomatic relief.

Corneal epithelial dystrophies

Corneal dystrophies are by definition bilateral, but may affect the two eyes asymmetrically. All are uncommon, except the map–dot–fingerprint (Cogan's microcystic) type, in which a variety of patterns (resembling maps, multiple dots, and fingerprints) can be seen in the epithelium of both corneas, particularly by retroillumination and scleral scatter illumination. Recurrent erosion is common, but the condition does not generally lead to significant visual impairment. Treat with lubricants, and bandage contact lens in severe cases.

Band keratopathy

Caused by calcium deposition in Bowman's membrane, in the interpalpebral cornea, which appears initially at the nasal and temporal limbus. It occurs in hypercalcaemia (hyperparathyroidism and sarcoid), following chronic ocular inflammation, total retinal detachment of longstanding, and in rubeotic eyes. Symptoms are caused by the visual effect of the calcium plaque in the visual axis, and sometimes by exposure of corneal nerves, causing pain. Plaques can be removed in symptomatic band keratopathy by excimer laser superficial keratectomy, or by chelation with topical EDTA under topical anaesthetic.

Stromal disease

Keratitis and corneal ulcer

Corneal inflammation is called keratitis; if this is complicated by stromal necrosis beneath an area of epithelial loss, the result is a corneal ulcer. The late effects of keratitis include neovascularization, lipid keratopathy, and scarring, which may seriously compromise vision, and require corneal graft. Grafting a vascularized cornea carries a high risk of failure due to rejection. The management of keratitis and corneal ulcer seeks to remove the contributing causes, and minimize tissue loss, inflammation, scarring, and vascularization.

Symptoms

Pain, impaired vision, photophobia, lacrimation, and discharge.

Signs

Ciliary injection, cellular infiltration, exudate, anterior uveitis, and corneal vascularization.

Aetiology

A combination of aetiological factors is usually responsible for the clinical picture in corneal ulcer. Bacterial infection may be the primary cause of the ulcer, or represent secondary superinfection. It is important that all the component factors associated with the development of an ulcer are identified (Table 3.1) and treated appropriately.

Assessment

1. Record accurately the size, shape, and depth of the ulcer, so that its progress and response to treatment, can be followed. (a) *Bacterial* ulcers are irregular with a ragged edge, filled with necrotic tissue and pus, and show

Table 3.1 Aetiology of corneal ulcer

Infective	bacterial
	primary or secondary
	viral (HSV)
	fungal
	amoebic (acanthamoeba)
Traumatic	abrasion
	foreign body
	burn
	chemical or thermal
	contact lens associated
	exposure
Inflammatory	vasculitic
	cornea alone
	systemic vasculitis (rheumatoid, Wegener's granuloma, PAN)
	marginal
	associated with staph. blepharitis
Nutritional	keratomalacia (vitamin A deficiency)
Degenerative	
Neurotrophic	V nerve damage
	herpes (simplex and zoster)
	leprosy
Contributory factors	
(a) Ocular	dry eye state
	lacrimal obstruction
	blepharitis
	bullous keratopathy
	trichiasis
	contact lens (especially extended-wear)
	corneal exposure
(b) General	immunosuppression
	diabetes
	rheumatoid
	alcoholism
	malnutrition
	extensive burns
	coma

marked surrounding inflammation and cellular infiltration. They are usually accompanied by purulent discharge, and cells in the anterior chamber, or hypopyon. (b) *Herpes simplex* produces a typically dendritic branching pattern, but may present with geographic (usually following topical steroids) or atypical ulcers. (c) *Neurotrophic* ulcers are clean, unless secondarily infected, and have a smooth irregular edge. The surrounding cornea has a dull glazed appearance. (d) *Fungal* keratitis occurs as an opportunist infection, or follows trauma from plant material (e.g. a thorn). There is a granular infiltrate in the anterior stroma, among which hyphae may be seen, but cellular infiltration is relatively slight. Surrounding microabscesses, 'satellite' lesions, or a ring abscess around the primary ulcer, are characteristic of fungal keratitis. The dull ulcer crater, its edges, or overlying epithelium, are often elevated above the surrounding cornea. (e) *Amoebic* keratitis presents with a painful epitheliopathy, typically with pseudodendrites or multiple erosions, infiltrates forming irregular patches, a ring or satellites, and scleritis. It usually occurs in contact lens wearers. (f) *Marginal* ulcers are round or oval, situated at the corneal margin, but often separated from the limbus by a clear zone, and commonly associated with a leash of episcleral and conjunctival vessels. (g) *Corneal melting* syndromes are characterized by progressive stromal lysis, extending centrally from a marginal gutter, in association with occlusive vasculopathy—particularly in conjunction with rheumatoid disease and Wegener's granulomatosis.

2. Test corneal sensation. Corneal sensation is particularly reduced (relative to the unaffected eye) in herpes simplex keratitis, because of V ganglion infection, and in amoebic keratitis. Neurotrophic ulcers occur in densely anaesthetic corneas, secondary to V nerve damage caused by tumour or surgery.

3. Take swabs and scrapes for Gram stain and culture, before applying local anaesthetic or fluorescein (these agents inhibit bacterial growth), and before treatment with antibiotics. Gram stain is important, since it not only gives an immediate indication of the type of organisms involved, and will indicate fungal aetiology, but also because many ulcers have already been treated with antibiotic before they reach an ophthalmologist, and culture often proves negative.

Treatment

Bacterial ulcers

Having taken swabs and scrapes, treat infected ulcers with intensive antibiotics and cycloplegia. In the first place treat according to Gram stain. If the infection is mixed, or Gram stain is unhelpful, use broad spectrum antibiotics, including anti-staphylococcal and anti-pseudomonas activity. These can be modified according to microbiological results if the clinical response is unsatisfactory. If microbiology has been negative and there is no clinical improvement, stop topical antibiotics for 24 h and then re-scrape and re-culture. Intensive concentrated antibiotic therapy may cause toxic epitheliopathy and delayed healing; this must be distinguished from failure of the infection to respond to therapy. Systemic therapy may be necessary if there is deep stromal involvement or perforation.

An appropriate initial regimen is:

- topical   concentrated antibiotic drops* half-hourly alternating: cefuroxime (37.5 mg/ml) (Gram positive); gentamicin (14 mg/ml) (Gram negative) atropine b.d.
- subconjunctival   mydricaine (atropine, adrenalin, procaine)
      subconjunctival antibiotics are only necessary if regular topical therapy is not possible.

If clinical response to the initial regime is poor, consider changing therapy to:

- pseudomonas   ticarcillin (50 mg/ml)
                                      tobramycin
- staph (pencillin sensitive)   benzyl pencillin (5000 u/ml)
                                      bacitracin
- staph (pencillin resistant)   vancomycin (50 mg/ml)
                                      methicillin (20 mg/ml)
                                      carbenicillin
                                      bacitracin
                                      flucloxacillin

Bacitracin and vancomycin may cause severe local reaction.

- *concentrated gentamicin drops: add 2 ml i.m./i.v. vial gentamicin (80 mg) to 5 ml of gentamicin eye drops (first remove 3 ml from 8 ml bottle, or 5 ml from 10 ml bottle). Final concentration = 14 mg/ml
- *concentrated cefuroxime drops: remove 1 ml from 10 ml bottle of hypromellose. Dilute 750 mg, i.m./i.v. cefuroxime in 2 ml saline. Add half of this to hypromellose bottle. Final concentration = 37.5 mg/ml

Concentrated cefuroxime has a shelf-life of 3 days if kept in a refrigerator, due to chemical instability.

Topical steroid may be necessary, to suppress inflammation and reduce final scarring, when the infection has responded to antibiotics. The timing, frequency and strength of steroid therapy in infective keratitis is a matter of fine judgement; steroid treatment may lead to rapid progression and perforation of a pseudomonas ulcer.

Viral ulcer
Dendritic herpes simplex (HSV) ulcer is best treated with oc. acyclovir five times a day until the epithelium has healed. Trifluorothymidine, vidarabine, cytosine arabinoside, and idoxuridine are alternative specific antivirals. Cytosine arabinoside is little used; idoxuridine has been superseded as the treatment of choice by acyclovir.

Debridement of infected epithelium is effective if specific antivirals are unavailable.

Steroids are absolutely contraindicated in epithelial herpes keratitis, since they facilitate viral replication, and predispose to geographic epithelial ulceration and stromal invasion.

Herpes simplex keratitis is more fully considered below.

Fungal ulcer
Satisfactory antifungal chemotherapy is less clearly established, partly because fungal ulcers are relatively uncommon.

Filamentous fungi (*Fusarium*, *Cephalosporium*, *Aspergillus*) infect traumatic ulcers involving plant material. Opportunist infections caused by yeasts (most often *Candida*), occur in corneas which are anaesthetic or neurotrophic, damaged (notably by HSV), or in debilitated or immunocompromised patients.

The principal antifungal agents used clinically are classed as polyenes, imidazole derivatives, and pyrimidines. Of these, there is most experience of topical treatment with:

1. *Polyenes*: (a) amphotericin B (0.5–10 mg/ml)—active against *Candida* and *Aspergillus*; (b) natamycin (50 mg/ml)—active against *Fusarium*.
2. *Imidazoles*: miconazole (10 mg/ml)—active against yeasts and some filamentous fungi.

Protozoal ulcer
Acanthamoeba causes a refractory destructive ulcer, often, but not always, associated with contact lens wear. It is treated with topical propamidine isethionate (brolene), neomycin, and steroid, but may require corneal grafting.

Neurotrophic ulcer
Basement membrane damage inhibits stable adhesion of the epithelium, and neurotrophic ulcers are chronic, indolent, difficult to heal, and at constant risk of secondary infection. They are treated by lubricants, tarsorrhaphy, or therapeutic bandage contact lens. A bandage lens carries the risk of drying and secondary infection, and must be used in conjunction with adequate artificial tear therapy, and monitored closely.

Rheumatoid and vascular (e.g. Mooren's) ulcers
Corneal necrosis is caused by local ischaemia (occlusive limbal vasculopathy) combined with lysis by collagenases (derived from leucocytes released from adjacent limbal and conjunctival vessels). These ulcers are a manifestation of systemic autoimmune disorder, usually rheumatoid or Wegener's granuloma. Treatment must therefore include systemic therapy, with steroids and in severe cases immunosuppression (cyclosporin A). Pulsed intravenous therapy (methylprednisolone 500 mg, i.v.) may help to arrest threatened perforation; this requires in-patient admission and appropriate monitoring. Topical steroids may contribute to suppression of the obliterative vasculitis, but also inhibit proliferation of fibroblasts and epithelial cells in the repair processes, and therefore may predispose to perforation. Acetylcysteine has some anticollagenase activity, and may limit stromal destruction.

Corneal scar
Scarring is the end stage of any corneal inflammation, and represents invasion of fibroblasts, often accompanied by blood vessels. Lipoprotein leak from corneal vessels leads to diffuse cloudiness of the adjacent stroma (lipid keratopathy).

Corneal scars are stable, but may cause considerable visual impairment if they are central. Treatment is by penetrating keratoplasty, or rotational autograft.

Corneal oedema

Optical clarity of the cornea depends upon its relative dehydration, which is maintained by the endothelial pump and evaporation-driven passage through the epithelium, which counterbalance the hydrating forces (IOP and colloid osmotic pressure of the stromal matrix). Endothelial disorder, or high elevation of IOP, cause decompensation and corneal oedema (bullous epitheliopathy and stromal thickening). Decompensation occurs at lower IOP in corneas in which endothelial function is already compromised by surgery or dystrophy.

Generalized oedema

Elevated IOP
- glaucoma (acute angle closure, rubeotic, or absolute),
- Posner–Schlossman syndrome.

Endothelial dysfunction
- surgery (especially cataract surgery with anterior chamber intraocular lens (IOL), or intracapsular extraction associated with vitreous-endothelial touch),
- keratitis (especially HSV, acanthamoeba),
- endothelial dystrophy,
- endothelial rejection (following penetrating graft).

Localized oedema
- disciform keratitis (HSV endotheliitis)
- keratoconus hydrops
- trauma (limited splits in Descemet's membrane)

Treatment

Treatment aims to resolve the reason for decompensation, or, if the eye is blind, is symptomatic.

Raised IOP
1. Topical antiglaucoma therapy, or oral acetazolamide. Beta-blockers are well-tolerated, but long-term acetazolamide is usually not.
2. Glaucoma surgery.

Irreversible endothelial cell loss
Penetrating keratoplasty is the only definitive solution if endothelial function is irreversibly compromised, in endothelial dystrophy, or following anterior segment surgery.

Symptomatic treatment
A bandage contact lens often relieves the pain caused by exposure of the corneal nerve endings due to rupture of epithelial bullae. Hypertonic (5 per cent) saline

ointment or drops sometimes clear a marginally decompensated cornea, and can be useful in relieving discomfort.

Herpes simplex keratitis (HSK)

Primary HSV infection is very common, giving rise to mild follicular blepharo-conjunctivitis during childhood, which may pass unnoticed. Following this the infection enters a latent phase in the trigeminal ganglion. Most clinical herpes simplex eye disease is secondary, the latent viruses passing along the nasociliary nerve (V_1) to re-invade the cornea.

Reactivation depends mainly on the virus strain, but also on host and environmental factors which are incompletely understood. Reinfection by a second exogenous HSV, once a primary colonization is established, probably only occurs in the immunocompromised. HSV causes epithelial, stromal, and endothelial disease, anterior uveitis, and (rarely) necrotizing retinitis.

HSK presents initially as a dendritic ulcer as virus replicates in epithelial cells. Epithelial extension produces a geographic ulcer, and invasion of the stroma initiates stromal keratitis: both these complications are facilitated by treatment of a dendritic ulcer with topical steroids. Disciform keratitis is a localized area of corneal oedema caused by reversible damage to the endothelium. Commonly the clinical picture is mixed. Anterior uveitis complicates any keratitis, including HSK; HS iritis also occurs without HSK. Corneal sensation is characteristically reduced in HSK and HS iritis.

Treatment of HSK requires an appreciation of the balance of four pathological processes: viral replication, host immune response, corneal anaesthesia and exposure, and secondary bacterial infection (Fig. 3.1).

Epithelial HSK

Uncomplicated dendritic ulcers are confined to the epithelium, and heal with only faint subepithelial scarring. Viral replication causes epithelial cell destruction, and is inhibited by acyclovir.

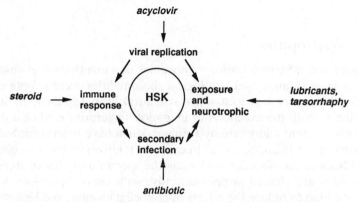

Fig. 3.1 The pathophysiology of herpes simplex keratitis.

Stromal keratitis

Destructive inflammation with ciliary injection, vascularization, cellular infiltration, necrosis and scarring, secondary anterior uveitis, and visual impairment. The principal pathology is an immune reaction to viral antigen in stroma. It is managed with acyclovir, topical steroid, and mydriatic, and treatment must be monitored closely. Stromal scarring due to HSK is the commonest cause of corneal blindness in the west, and a common indication for penetrating keratoplasty.

Disciform keratitis

A localized area of corneal oedema, with localized KP and mild anterior chamber reaction, intact epithelium and no signs of stromal inflammation. Caused by focal endothelial dysfunction, due to antigen–antibody effects on the endothelial cells. Responds to treatment with topical steroids over 7–10 days.

Metaherpetic keratitis

Tear film abnormalities combine with corneal anaesthesia to produce neurotrophic ulcers. These are shapeless ulcers with irregular edges, associated with low-grade surrounding cellular infiltration of the stroma. The corneal surface is densely anaesthetic and appears lacklustre. Treatment is aimed at protecting the epithelial environment, with artificial tears, bandage contact lens, and tarsorrhaphy.

Herpes simplex anterior uveitis

The KP are translucent and globular, resembling 'baconfat', and there is characteristic sector atrophy of the iris, seen best on transillumination. Treatment is with topical steroid and mydriatic to prevent scarring, while monitoring the cornea to avoid facilitating HSK. Acyclovir (ACV) cover should be added if there is a possibility of epithelial disease.

Corneal dystrophies

Dystrophies are inherited (mostly autosomal dominant) corneal disorders in which specific anatomical and histological abnormalities occur in both eyes, and are confined more or less to a single structural layer (epithelium, stroma or endothelium). With the exception of map–dot–fingerprint epithelial dystrophy they are uncommon; many rare dystrophies which have been recorded will not be described here. It can be useful to examine relatives in order to confirm the inherited basis of the disorder, and study the spectrum of clinical signs.

Dystrophies are treated symptomatically, with tinted spectacles to reduce glare, lubrication to reduce the effects of epithelial erosion, and by keratoplasty if necessary for visual reasons.

Epithelial dystrophies

Map–dot–fingerprint (Cogan's microcystic)

Irregular patches of epithelial cloudiness, the topography of which may be whorled, linear, or geographic, and is changeable. The cloudiness is due to intraepithelial cysts containing cellular debris, and the linear features are associated with folding of the basement membrane. Map–dot–fingerprint dystrophy is often associated with recurrent corneal erosion, but seldom causes significant visual symptoms. Treatment is symptomatic, with artificial tears for lubrication, or bandage contact lens. Epithelial debridement has been suggested where recurrent erosion is particularly troublesome.

Meesman's

Microcysts in the corneal epithelium, present from the first year of life, and increasing progressively in number thereafter. Symptoms begin during adulthood, when the cysts, diffusely distributed throughout the entire corneal epithelium, rupture from time to time and cause recurrent erosions. Attempts to cure Meesman's by keratoplasty are usually followed by recurrence in the graft.

Reis–Bücklers'

Presents during childhood with recurrent central erosions, which cause discomfort, photophobia, and lacrimation. The central cornea becomes cloudy, with an irregular surface and irregular astigmatism, as the disorder progresses in adulthood, and stabilizes in middle age. Penetrating keratoplasty may then be undertaken, but recurrences in the graft have been reported.

Stromal dystrophies

Granular

Fine granules in the anterior cornea, which progressively spread throughout the cornea, sparing its periphery, and coalesce into an amorphous reticulum. The granules have characteristic histological and electron microscopic (EM) characteristics, although their origin is not known. Though they may give rise to troublesome glare, keratoplasty is seldom necessary.

Macular

A very uncommon, but severe dystrophy, which is recessively inherited. The superficial cornea is initially diffusely hazy, the opacities aggregating by early adulthood to form dense masses or nodules throughout the cornea, together with central thinning. The underlying disorder is probably an abnormality of keratan (corneal glycosaminoglycan) synthesis. Penetrating keratoplasty is necessary to restore vision, but macular deposits may recur in the graft.

Lattice

A reticulum of fine refractile lines, initially in the superficial and middle layers of the cornea, associated with recurrent erosions. Corneal sensation is often progressively impaired, and sometimes the opacities, which are composed of amyloid, may become sufficiently dense to require corneal graft.

Endothelial dystrophies

Cornea guttata and Fuchs'

Progressive reduction of endothelial capacity, leading ultimately, in severe cases, to spontaneous corneal decompensation and oedema, followed by scarring. Most cases do not progress beyond the stage of guttata, in which scattered brown deposits are seen on the endothelium, associated with an endothelial *peau d'orange* appearance on specular illumination under high magnification. Corneas with guttata are at risk of decompensation following minimal surgical trauma, or on modest elevations of intraocular pressure, and peroperative clouding may compromise the surgeon's view during cataract surgery. Irreversible decompensation is treated by penetrating keratoplasty.

Posterior polymorphous

Opacities of variable size, morphology, density, and interocular symmetry, associated with progressive thickening of Descemet's membrane, and often with congenital iridocorneal anomalies in the angle, evident on gonioscopy. If these are extensive, the condition may be complicated by glaucoma. Abnormal differentiation of the neural crest mesoderm cells during angle cleavage may account for the abnormal endothelial cell behaviour in posterior polymorphous dystrophy. Decompensation is unusual, but may require penetrating keratoplasty.

Keratoconus (KC)

KC is an ectasia of the central cornea, caused by stromal thinning, which leads to the normally spherical anterior corneal face becoming conical, with consequent degradation of the retinal image. It presents usually during teenage years, is commoner in atopic patients, and is often bilateral, but asymmetric. There is a high incidence of KC in Down's syndrome, in whom the onset is characteristically early.

Diagnosis

- swirling irregular retinoscopy reflex,
- irregular astigmatism,
- keratoscopy (irregular reflection of mires),
- Fleischer ring (epithelial pigment ring at cone edge),
- Munson's sign (indentation of lower lid margin on down-gaze),
- Vogt's striae (fine folds in Descemet's membrane, approximating to cone's long axis),
- fine streaks in anterior stroma,
- Placido's disc (irregular reflection of circular image).

Clinical course

The rate of progressive enlargement of the cone is variable. Rapid progression leads to tears in Descemet's membrane, and acute focal decompensation and oedema — 'hydrops'. Eyes with hydrops must be carefully watched, in case infection or perforation occur, though these complications are uncommon, and hydrops generally resolves leaving a degree of stromal scarring.

Management

Hard contact lens
This corrects the irregular corneal refracting surface, and restores good vision, until the cone is too steep to permit contact lens stability (K > 50D–60D), when penetrating keratoplasty must be considered.

Penetrating graft
This replaces the cone with a normal donor cornea in advanced KC, when contact lens correction has become impossible due to lens instability, or following resolution of hydrops.

Metabolic corneal disorders

Lipid keratopathy

Lipid deposition is associated with corneal neovascularization following inflammation or trauma. It must be distinguished (using slit-lamp examination at high magnification) from active infiltration by inflammatory cells.

Arcus senilis

Arcus senilis is a symmetrical peripheral deposition of lipid. If present in presenile eyes it indicates a disorder of lipid metabolism, which should be investigated biochemically.

Band keratopathy

Calcium salts accumulating at the level of Bowman's membrane, in a band distribution corresponding to the palpebral aperture, associated with chronic inflammation or calcium metabolic disorder.

Kayser–Fleischer ring

A greenish-brown ring in the peripheral part of Descemet's membrane. It occurs in Wilson's disease (caused by defective copper transport associated with ceruloplasmin deficiency), together with nystagmus and generalized choreiform movement disorder, and cirrhosis.

Inherited disorders of metabolism

Certain unusual inherited disorders feature corneal clouding.

Mucopolysaccharidoses
Hurler's disease, Scheie's syndrome: associated dysmorphism.

Mucolipidoses (MLS)
MLS I–IV: associated with variable mental, psychomotor, and growth disorders.

Sphingolipidoses
Metachromatic leucodystrophy, Fabry's disease: vortex keratopathy, renal failure, neuropathy.

Cystinosis
Intrastromal crystal deposits. Infantile cystinosis is associated with severe nephropathy.

Sclera and episclera

Episcleritis
Episcleritis is usually an isolated local condition, causing mild pricking or aching discomfort. There is diffuse or nodular episceleral injection, without intraocular inflammation or visual impairment. It can be distinguished from conjunctivitis by gently moving a moist cotton-wool bud over the anaesthetized conjunctiva at the slit-lamp: conjunctival vessels move, while episceral vessels do not.

Treatment is symptomatic, with topical steroids to relieve discomfort.

Scleritis (see p. 123)
Scleritis commonly occurs as part of systemic inflammatory disorder, particularly rheumatoid and Wegener's granulomatosis.

Clinical features
Scleritis presents with severe boring pain radiating to the forehead, and marked tenderness on palpation and pressure; vision is often impaired, due to macular oedema. Examine the affected sclera in daylight with the lids well-retracted — it is thickened, red (brawny), and tender. Slit-lamp examination may show uveitis, serous retinal detachment, and macular oedema. There may also be proptosis and limitation of eye movement. Scleral necrosis may lead to thinning (scleromalacia perforans) and risk of rupture.

Ultrasonic signs (using combined B- and vector A-scan) are useful in diagnosis and assessment of response to treatment.

1. The posterior coats of the healthy eye have a thickness of less than 2 mm; this may be increased to as much as 10 mm in scleritis.
2. In scleritis there is a lucent zone behind the thickened posterior sclera, which is caused by accumulation of episcleral oedema fluid.

Management
There is usually underlying systemic inflammatory disorder (rheumatoid, Wegener's granuloma, or chronic sepsis). This requires appropriate investigation and management in conjunction with a rheumatologist. The underlying pathology is probably an immune-mediated occlusive vasculitis, and treatment

requires systemic steroids, in high dose initially (100 mg prednisolone, re-ducing according to clinical response), or intermittent ('pulsed') injections of intravenous methylprednisolone. Immunosuppression with cyclosporin may be necessary.

Complications of scleritis are due to involvement of adjacent structures in the inflammatory process: keratitis, uveitis, secondary glaucoma, cataract, cystoid macular oedema, serous retinal detachment, and optic neuritis.

Lens

Anatomy

The lens contains protein (α- and β-crystallin) fibres, which are the accumulated remnants of capsule cells. These cells migrate inwards from the mitotic zone at the equator, lose their nucleus, and become flattened. There is a layer of lens epithelial cells on the inner surface of the anterior lens capsule, but not on the thinner posterior capsule. As the lens ages, its nucleus becomes progressively more dense and hard (nuclear sclerosis), and may accumulate a brown pigment. Together with loss of transparency due to vacuolation and regional failure of dehydration, these increasing optical imperfections contribute to senile cataract formation. Until the age of 30–40 years the contents of the lens capsule can be aspirated, but above this age the nucleus is hard, and can only be removed by extraction or phacoemulsification.

The lens is suspended at its equator from the ciliary body by the zonule. Zonular fibres are continuous with the lens capsule and fibres of the ciliary body stroma. They transmit tension in the ciliary body to the capsule, and thus influence the shape of the lens, and therefore its converging power.

Physiology

The optical transparency of the lens depends upon a constant state of relative dehydration, and preservation of the tertiary structure of its proteins. These are maintained by glycolytic metabolic activity in the lens cell membranes, driving Ca^{2+}-dependent Na^+–K^+ ion pumps. Any disturbance in this equilibrium may lead to loss of transparency.

The young lens assumes a more spherical shape when tension on the radial zonular fibres is reduced by circular ciliary muscle contraction: its dioptric power then increases (accommodation). Older lenses have a diminished ability to deform, and therefore a reduced accommodative range (presbyopia).

Cycloplegia blocks the parasympathetic innervation to the circular ciliary muscle and abolishes accommodation. Mydriasis (relaxation of the iris sphincter) inevitably accompanies pharmacologically induced cycloplegia, but can be achieved with minimal cycloplegia (for lens and posterior segment examination) using tropicamide.

The lens responds to most insults by becoming cloudy. It may also become subluxated or dislocated, and it occasionally exhibits congenital defects.

Congenital lens abnormalities

Coloboma of the lens is uncommon, and is usually accompanied by iris coloboma.

Congenital cataract is often inherited; it may be associated with intrauterine disorder, or persistent hyperplastic primary vitreous.

Congenital dislocation is most commonly inherited, and may be associated with metabolic disorder.

The management of congenital lens disorders is discussed in Chapter 10.

Cataract

Loss of clarity of the lens which causes impairment of visual function is called cataract. The visual requirement of patients, and therefore the stage at which cataract becomes sufficiently troublesome to warrant extraction, varies enormously.

Aetiology

The principal aetiological associations of cataract are listed in Table 3.2.

Most cataracts are associated with ageing; the specific biochemical changes causing these cataracts are not clear. A biochemical aetiology has been proposed in cataract associated with some metabolic disorders, especially those involving sugar and calcium metabolism. The cause of cataract following chronic ocular inflammation is not clearly established, and traumatic cataract is probably caused by damage to the anterior capsular cells.

Assessment

Establish the extent that visual disability caused by lens opacities interferes with the patient's activities. Two important questions must be answered:

1. To what extent is visual impairment caused by cataract?
2. To what extent is the patient inconvenienced by poor vision due to cataract?

Table 3.2   Cataract — aetiological associations

Congenital	idiopathic
	intrauterine infection (rubella, toxoplasma, cytomegalovirus, HSV)
	chromosome abnormality
	metabolic (diabetes, calcium, galactose)
Acquired	idiopathic senile
	metabolic (diabetes, calcium, Wilson's disease)
	trauma (physical, radiation)
	inflammation (uveitis, Fuchs' heterochromic iridocyclitis)
	steroid induced
	dermatopathy
	retinitis pigmentosa
	dystrophia myotonica

Symptoms

It is very important that the patient describes the nature of any visual impairment. There may be little or none in unilateral cataract, and in patients with limited visual requirements. The location of the opacity within the lens determines the symptoms it causes (see below).

Amblyopia (history of lazy or weak eye since childhood, or squint) causes acuity loss which will not be corrected by cataract surgery. Patients are usually aware that one eye has 'always been weak'.

Onset of visual loss is gradual in cataract (except following trauma, loss of vision occurs over weeks, months, or years). Sudden visual loss is not due to cataract, though gradual loss may be noticed fortuitously and thought to be sudden.

Examination

Visual acuity

Test acuity unaided, with spectacle correction, and following refraction if the spectacle correction is not recent. Clinical Snellen testing indicates acuity under optimal conditions, and considerably underestimates the visual impairment caused by glare, especially in anterior cortical cataract. Add −1 DS to assess whether induced myopia caused by nuclear sclerosis can be improved by changed spectacle correction.

Retinoscopy reflex

The brightness of the retinoscopy reflex, and opacities within it, give a good idea of the clarity of optical transmission through the lens. Discrepancy between the reflexes of the two eyes compared with their acuities may suggest that lens opacities do not entirely account for the observed acuities.

Relative afferent pupil test

Negative relative afferent pupil defect excludes optic nerve disorder as a cause of the visual loss. Relative afferent pupil defect in patients under consideration for cataract surgery is most commonly due to anterior ischaemic optic neuropathy or advanced glaucoma. Cataract surgery will be of little benefit to these patients.

Slit-lamp examination

This reveals the density and distribution of lens opacities. The lens should be examined at the slit-lamp following dilation, since adequate assessment may be impossible through a small pupil.

Posterior segment examination through a dilated pupil

This is necessary to exclude retinal or macular pathology. Examine the entire fundus with the indirect ophthalmoscope, and the macula, disc, and vessels with the 90D lens at the slit-lamp. It can sometimes be difficult to reconcile objective signs of macular disorder with visual acuity.

Morphological–aetiological–clinical correlations

Posterior subcapsular cataract
This is associated with chronic and recurrent anterior uveitis, chronic topical or systemic steroid therapy, and retinitis pigmentosa. It causes marked impairment of acuity even though most of the lens substance is clear, since the opacity is located near the nodal point of the eye.

Anterior cortical cataract
This may appear very dense at the slit-lamp, while allowing surprisingly good acuity under good lighting conditions. Direct light (oncoming traffic headlamps or low sun) causes disabling glare.

Nuclear sclerosis (often with a central brown opacity)
This occurs in senile cataract, and is associated with myopic shift in refraction. Correction of this may significantly improve distance vision.

Cortical spokes
These radiate from the periphery to the centre and are characteristic of diabetic cataract. Vision is impaired when the centre of the lens becomes involved.

Lamellar cataract
This implies a biochemical or inflammatory cause occurring during a finite period *in utero* or early infancy.

Indications for surgery

Cataract extraction is indicated if significant improvement in visual function would follow surgery. The decision to operate is based on an assessment that lens opacities are responsible for visual impairment, which is causing significant inconvenience or difficulty. It therefore involves a judgement by both ophthalmologist and patient, and the indications for surgery differ from one patient to another.

Surgery to a second eye may provide little improvement in binocular acuity, but improves stereopsis, especially at near, and widens the visual field. It is generally not undertaken within 3 months of the first.

Cataract surgery is not contraindicated by maculopathy. The improvement in navigating vision may be very useful, but the patients should be warned that the clarity of central ('detailed') vision may not improve.

Cataract extraction under local anaesthesia is very satisfactory; there are no anaesthetic contraindications to surgery.

Correction of aphakia

The optical difficulties posed by the correction of aphakia (especially following unilateral cataract extraction) are overcome most satisfactorily by the use of intraocular lenses (IOLs). There are few contraindications to IOL implantation, and posterior chamber IOLs are associated with very low morbidity. The appropriate IOL power is calculated preoperatively by computing axial length and anterior corneal curve on a nomogram.

Aphakic correction with spectacle lenses is accompanied by optical problems (image magnification causing diplopia, distortion, and peripheral field loss). Contact lenses avoid some of these problems, but are difficult for many patients to manage.

IOLs in infants and children present particular problems (the growth of the eye, refractive change and the prevention of amblyopia). Most surgeons do not use them in infants, and their use in children, and the minimum age at which it is safe to implant an IOL, are matters of debate. However, IOLs are now routinely used in younger patients than was formerly the case, as the low morbidity associated with their use becomes clear.

Following cataract surgery order the final pseudophakic correction about 2 months postoperatively. If there is an astigmatic error greater than 2 DC divide or remove the sutures (in the axis of the + cylinder) after 8 weeks, and refract finally a month later.

Ectopic lens

Aetiology

- congenital,
- hereditary,
- traumatic,
- Marfan's syndrome,
- Weil–Marchesani syndrome,
- homocystinuria,
- Treacher Collins syndrome.

Presentation

- astigmatism,
- diplopia,
- iridodonesis,
- low-grade uveitis,
- glaucoma.

Children presenting with ectopia should be investigated to identify or exclude metabolic causes.

Management

Surgical removal of an ectopic lens is technically difficult, requiring vitrectomy instrumentation, and may be complicated. Ectopia is best managed conservatively if possible, by optimizing vision, and managing glaucoma and uveitis appropriately.

Recommended further reading

Harding, J. (1991). *Cataract. Biochemistry, epidemiology and pharmacology*. Chapman and Hall, London.

Jaffe, N.S., Jaffe, M.S., and Jaffe, G.F. (1990). *Cataract surgery and its complications*, 5th edn. Mosby, St Louis.

Kaufman, Barron, McDonald, and Waltman. (1988). *The cornea*. Churchill Livingstone, New York.

Watson, P.G. and Hazelman, B.L. (1976). *The sclera and systemic disorders*. W.B. Saunders, London.

4

The posterior segment

The structures behind the lens constitute the posterior segment. Disorders of the posterior segment give rise to visual symptoms without external signs, apart from the afferent pupil defect, which is positive if there is optic nerve disease or extensive loss of retinal function.

The posterior segment comprises the vitreous, the retina (including the macula) and its vessels, the retinal pigment epithelium, Bruch's membrane and the choroid, the posterior sclera, and the optic nerve head.

The fundus is the part of the eye seen with an ophthalmoscope. It comprises:

1. *The posterior pole*. The central area, within the temporal vessel arcades. The macula is located within the central retina.

2. *The equator*. The equator corresponds to the meridian of the eye's greatest transverse diameter, lying between the periphery and the posterior pole. In this zone the retinal vessels branch from the four major arcades. Diabetic retinal neovascularization usually appears earliest in the equatorial retina.

3. *The periphery*. The most anterior part of the fundus, seen best with the indirect ophthalmoscope using indentation, or by three-mirror examination at the slit-lamp. The retina ends at the ora serrata, behind the pars plana of the ciliary body. Peripheral retina is thin, with fine vessels, and is subject to degeneration and tears.

Disorders affecting the posterior segment can conveniently be considered as involving the retina and its vessels, the subretinal tissues, the macula, the disc, and the vitreoretinal complex (including retinal detachment).

Examination

Examine the posterior segment through a dilated pupil, using the indirect and direct ophthalmoscope, and the slit-lamp in conjunction with accessory lenses. Each method provides an image which is useful for particular aspects of examination.

The indirect ophthalmoscope gives a wide binocular view, which extends to the ora serrata (using indentation), at low magnification ($\times$ 6). It gives an overall perspective for initial examination, showing the four vessel arcades simultaneously, and is particularly useful in the examination of retinal detachment and identification of retinal breaks, and to provide a comparative view of the two fundi. Because of its extended depth of focus, abnormalities of the vitreous are best seen with the indirect.

The slit-lamp is used for magnified three-dimensional biomicroscopy of the fundus. Because of its short focal length, accessory lenses must be used. Biomicroscopy is particularly useful for three-dimensional examination of the macula, to define thickening and oedema, and the disc, to show cupping and disc vessels. The 90D and 78D lenses give an inverted image, the Hruby lens gives an erect image, and the Goldmann three-mirror contact lens gives an erect image of the posterior pole through its central lens, and a laterally inverted image of the equator and periphery through its prisms.

The direct ophthalmoscope gives a monocular view at high magnification (× 16), and may be used to examine details of the disc, macula and vessels, and other structures of interest seen with the indirect.

4(a)   RETINA

Retinal anatomy

The neuroretina has an outer layer of receptors (rods and cones), whose cell bodies synapse with the bipolar cells; these in turn project to the ganglion cells whose axons course across the surface of the retina as the nerve fibre layer to reach the optic disc, where they form the optic nerve. The synapses between successive retinal layers are complex, with lateral as well as vertical organization; the complexity of retinal architecture is increased by the horizontal and amacrine cells (whose function is not well understood) and Müller's cells.

The layers of the neuroretina are differentiated histologically into the receptor layer, outer nuclear (receptor cell bodies), outer plexiform (receptor–bipolar synapses), inner nuclear (bipolar cells), inner plexiform (bipolar–ganglion cell connections), the ganglion cell layer, and finally the nerve fibre layer. The footplates of Müller's cells insert into the internal limiting membrane, which lies internal to the nerve fibre layer and forms the outer boundary of the vitreous.

The retinal pigment epithelium (RPE) is a single layer of non-replicating pigment cells, whose function includes phagocytosis of the receptor plates, and metabolism and recycling of receptor pigments in the rhodopsin cycle. It is separated from the choroid externally by Bruch's membrane, a fibrous and elastic sheet which includes the basement membranes of RPE and choroid.

Retinal blood supply

The central retinal artery enters the optic nerve a few millimetres behind the eye, and divides first into superior and inferior branches, and then into nasal and temporal branches, each supplying a quadrant of the retina. Retinal veins follow the same pattern. The major arcades lie on the surface of the retina, giving a superficial capillary plexus which communicates with a deep plexus in the inner plexiform layer. Tissues deeper than the inner nuclear layer derive metabolic support by diffusion from the choroidal circulation via the RPE.

A cilioretinal artery emerges from the temporal margin of the disc in 20 per cent of individuals to supply the nasal part of the macula; it is derived from the posterior ciliary vessels, and unlike the retinal artery and its branches is vulnerable to giant cell arteritis. It must be distinguished from its (pathological) venous counterpart, the opticociliary shunt (a collateral venous channel which may open in the presence of progressive compression of the retrobulbar optic nerve by nerve sheath meningioma).

Retinal capillaries differ from most other capillaries in having tight junctions between their continuous layer of endothelial cells, and they are surrounded by pericytes with an external basement membrane. Retinal capillaries are much less permeable than other capillaries, and there are no retinal lymphatics. Abnormal leakage occurs in diabetic retinopathy, inflammation, and trauma, and causes retinal oedema which severely impairs retinal function.

Signs of retinal disorder

Haemorrhage

The shape of retinal haemorrhages defines their level within the retina:

• Flame shaped (nerve fibre layer, NFL)	The course of nerve fibres in superficial retina can be seen. NFL haemorrhages derive from superficial capillary leaks.
• Blot (intraretinal)	Confined by retinal tissue. Intraretinal haemorrhages follow retinal vein occlusion, and if large, dark, and associated with cotton wool spots (CWS), imply ischaemia. Large, deep, dark, irregular haemorrhages are located deep within the retina and imply extensive ischaemia.

Subretinal haemorrhages are dark and smooth-edged. They usually occur beneath the macula, due to bleeding from a subretinal neovascular membrane (SRNVM), and may cause elevation or oedema of the overlying retina. Subretinal haemorrhage may also complicate drainage of subretinal fluid during retinal detachment surgery.

Exudate

Hard exudates (HE) represent the lipid remnants of long-term leak of plasma after resorption of fluid and proteins. Leaks from retinal vessels cause accumulation of HE in mid and superficial retina, while deep or subretinal HE derive from subretinal vessels. Their size, shape, and distribution are variable. A circinate pattern of exudate derives from a leak at their centre, while diffuse leak from the area of the disc leads to a 'macular star' (due to accumulation of HE in the radiating axons of macular ganglion cells in Henlé's layer).

Retinal oedema

Retinal oedema (thickening) represents continuing active leak, with fluid accumulation. This is seen on slit-lamp biomicroscopy and fluorescein angiography.

Cotton wool spots (CWS)

CWS are areas of opaque nerve fibre layer swelling, caused by ischaemia: axoplasmic flow is interrupted distal to the ischaemic focus, leading to focal accumulation of mitochondria within nerve fibres. Multiple CWS imply widespread ischaemia, and threat of neovascular proliferation.

Vessels

Abnormal retinal vessels may represent neovascular proliferation, anastamosis, or angiogenic tumour.

Neovascularization

New vessels (NV) are a proliferative vascular response to retinal ischaemia. They are fine, spidery vessels which grow in trails, fronds, or rosettes. Deficient endothelial integrity causes leakage (shown on fluorescein angiography), and deficient mural cell integrity leads to rupture and haemorrhage. Neovascularization is the hallmark of proliferative diabetic retinopathy, and occurs in conjunction with variable parallel fibroblastic stimulation.

- NVD = NV at the optic disc,
- NVE = NV elsewhere,
- NVF = NV forward from the retinal vascular plane, which are especially
       vulnerable to shearing, rupture, and haemorrhage.

Intraretinal microvascular abnormalities (IRMA)

IRMA are foci of fine intraretinal vessel complexes in diabetic retinopathy, which indicate retinal ischaemia and represent an early stage of endothelial proliferation.

Microaneurysms

Another component of diabetic retinopathy, microaneurysms (ma) appear as fine red dots, often in clumps. Focal weakness and dilatation of diabetic retinal capillary walls is caused by defective pericytes and hyaline accumulation in the basement membrane. Leakage from ma causes exudation of fluid and lipid, giving rise to a zone of oedema, and hard exudates which sometimes have a circinate pattern. Ruptured ma produce small retinal haemorrhages.

Collateral vessels

Collaterals are alternative vascular channels which bypass focal vessel obstruction. Vessels running from superotemporal retinal capillaries to the inferotemporal vein following superotemporal branch vein occlusion, or from distal superior temporal branch vein around an occlusion to proximal superotemporal branch vein, are collaterals.

Collateral channels derive from dilated capillaries. They are fine and convoluted, can be traced from the involved retina to patent veins, and show no leakage on fluorescein angiography.

Shunts

Shunts are abnormal vessels passing from arteries to veins, bypassing the capillary bed. Microvascular shunts occur as adaptations to capillary bed closure in diabetic retinopathy. Racemose haemangiomas (Wyburn–Mason syndrome) and retinal angiomas in von Hippel–Lindau's disease are examples of congenital shunts.

Sheathing

Vessel sheathing follows vasculitis, occurring in some autoimmune inflammatory disorders including systemic lupus erythematosus, sarcoid, and Behçet's disease. Sensitization to retinal antigens, which are normally isolated from the immune system, may play a part in the pathogenesis.

Occluded branch veins sometimes become sheathed.

Drusen

Drusen are discrete pale yellowish subretinal bodies, with a smooth outline, occurring with increasing frequency over the age of 50 years. They are located at the level of Bruch's membrane, may cause overlying RPE atrophy, give rise to window defect hyperfluorescence on fluorescein angiography, and are sometimes associated with SRNVM.

They represent an accumulation of photoreceptor metabolic by-products, which are normally transported through RPE and across Bruch's membrane to be removed by the choroidal circulation. Drusen are distinguished from HE by their more regular size and shape, less bright appearance (because they are subretinal), and regular bilateral distribution.

Vascular retinopathies

Retinal vascular disorders occur in association with hypertension and arteriopathy, diabetes, and certain systemic inflammatory disorders. The retina is damaged by ischaemia, leakage, and haemorrhage, due to changes in the blood vessel walls. Similar pathology elsewhere, especially cerebrovascular and renal disease, is common. The treatment of these disorders includes management of their systemic aspects.

Amaurosis fugax

Transient reversible painless loss of vision in one eye, lasting from 1 to 10 min, is the retinal analogue of a transient ischaemic attack in the cerebral circulation.

It is caused by atheromatous or platelet microembolization, usually derived from the carotid tree or the heart; the emboli may sometimes be seen in the retinal arterioles. Visual loss or recovery often occurs in an altitudinal pattern. It indicates serious carotid atherosclerosis, and the patient should be examined for carotid bruit or cardiac arrhythmia. Referral should be made to a physician for management, since anticoagulation or endarterectomy may be necessary.

Hypertensive retinopathy

Hypertension and arteriosclerosis commonly coexist. Both contribute to vessel and retinal damage, and the signs of hypertensive retinopathy: vessel wall thickening, leakage and exudate, haemorrhage, retinal ischaemia, and ischaemia papillopathy (Table 4.1).

Table 4.1 Clinical signs of retinopathy in hypertension and arteriosclerosis

	Arteriosclerotic	Hypertensive
Grade 1	copper wire reflex	vessel attenuation
Grade 2	silver wire reflex focal constriction	irregular vessel calibre,
Grade 3	mild AV nipping	haemorrhages, exudates, few CWS
Grade 4	severe AV nipping	severe grade 3 signs + CWS + disc oedema

Treatment of hypertensive retinopathy is directed at the hypertension. Grade 4 hypertensive retinopathy occurs in accelerated hypertension, which requires immediate referral to a physician.

Retinal artery occlusion

Atheromatous, cholesterol, or platelet emboli may occlude any branch of the carotoid tree, including the central retinal, or a branch retinal artery. Ischaemic retina in the territory of the occluded vessel becomes pale and swollen, with empty vessels.

Central retinal artery occlusion (CRAO) causes sudden painless complete loss of vision, with relative afferent pupil defect (RAPD). The entire retina is pale, because of oedema, while the macula is highlighted as a cherry red spot (because the underlying choroid shows through the thinner foveal retina). The macula may be partially spared by a cilioretinal vessel. Treatment by immediate paracentesis to reduce the intraocular pressure (IOP) drastically sometimes restores the retinal circulation, if it can be performed within an hour or two of the occlusion. Medical measures to reduce IOP and ocular massage are usually undertaken but are seldom effective.

Retinal vein occlusion

Central retinal vein occlusion (CRVO)

Signs
- retinal haemorrhages (NFL and intraretinal) in all four quadrants,
- dilated, tortuous veins,
- retinal thickening,
- disc swelling,
- CWS signify retinal ischaemia.

Ischaemic CRVO predisposes to anterior segment neovascularization (rubeosis). New vessels proliferate from the pupil margin to cover the iris and involve the drainage angle, causing rubeotic glaucoma. Rubeosis is resistant to medical and conventional surgical treatment, and is best prevented by early panretinal photocoagulation (PRP) of CRVO with ischaemia signs; PRP sometimes reverses early established rubeosis. Tube and plate drainage surgery has limited success in rubeotic eyes. A blind, painful rubeotic eye is best treated symptomatically with atropine and steroid drops.

Predisposing conditions
- ocular: glaucoma;
- vascular: inflammatory (vasculitis), hypertension;
- haematological: hyperviscosity, polycythaemia, clotting abnormality.

Papillophlebitis

A variant of CRVO, papillophlebitis ('incipient central retinal vein occlusion') occurs typically in young females (20–40 years old). It presents with a swollen disc and engorged dilated veins but with few retinal haemorrhages and no exudates, CWS or other signs of ischaemia, and good vision. Papillophlebitis has a benign course, resolving spontaneously after 1–6 months without permanent visual loss. Its cause is not known.

Branch retinal vein occlusion (BRVO)

BRVO occurs usually at a proximal AV crossing on the upper or lower temporal vessel arcade.

Signs
- distal to the occlusion: retinal haemorrhages (intraretinal and NFL), venous dilatation and tortuosity;
- variable macular oedema.

Collateral vessels open after some weeks, either around the occlusion to a patent proximal segment of the occluded vein, or across the horizontal midline to the other temporal arcade. A macular tributary vein may be selectively occluded, causing macular oedema with few haemorrhages.

Complications and treatment
Retinal neovascularization complicates BRVO with ischaemia (indicated by CWS, and capillary dropout on fluorescein angiography). If there are significant signs of ischaemia, sector PRP should be applied to the affected quadrant to prevent neovascularization. Macular grid laser therapy may be effective in reducing macular oedema.

It is important to distinguish collaterals from neovascularization, since NV must be eliminated by sector PRP and direct ablation; closure of collaterals further compromises the adaptations made by the retinal circulation, and exacerbates retinal oedema.

Diabetic retinopathy (DR)

Pathology

Retinal damage in diabetes is caused by:
• increased vessel permeability (abnormal endothelial cells),
• weakened vessel walls (decreased pericytes and thickened basement membrane),
• decreased blood flow (increased glycosylated haemoglobin),
• vascular occlusion,
• fibrovascular proliferation.

These processes cause:

• serum exudate leading to oedema and intraretinal lipid accumulation,
• ischaemia,
• haemorrhage,
• traction retinal detachment.

The haemodynamic changes underlying diabetic retinopathy result from decreased blood flow due to a combination of vessel wall thickening, increased blood viscosity, and red cell rigidity. The capillary basement membrane accumulates hyaline and becomes thickened, pericyte numbers are reduced, and the junctions between endothelial cells become incompetent. Simultaneously, increased glycosylation of red blood cell haemoglobin increases resistance to blood flow. The result is luminal narrowing, focal dilatation, reduced blood flow and leakage, leading to ischaemia, haemorrhage, and exudation.

The two pathways by which sight is damaged in diabetes are:

1. *Neovascularization.* Ischaemic retina stimulates proliferation of new vessels and fibrous membranes. The new vessels bleed, especially as they are torn from the retina during separation of the posterior vitreous, leading to retrohyaloid or vitreous haemorrhage. Contraction of the fibrous element of a fibrovascular membrane causes traction retinal detachment; if a retinal break occurs the detachment gains a rhegmatogenous component.

2. *Diabetic maculopathy.* The macula is damaged by a variable combination of ischaemia, oedema, accumulation of hard exudate and haemorrhage.

Diabetic retinopathy is a dynamic process, in which capillary narrowing (producing ischaemia response) is followed by focal or regional capillary closure (terminating the ischaemic response). Similarly, leakage from any source ceases when the lumen of a microaneurysm is occluded, or its capillary supply closes off.

Classification

Classification of DR

1. *Background*. Retinal haemorrhages (NFL and small blot), microaneurysms, IRMA, and hard exudates which pose no foveal threat. All background retinopathy changes are intraretinal.

2. *Pre-proliferative*. Background retinopathy with additional signs of ischaemia: more than six CWS, multiple large IRMA, venous beading, sausaging, reduplication, large deep dark haemorrhages.

3. *Proliferative*. Active neovascularization: new vessels at the disc (NVD), new vessels forward into the vitreous (NVF), new vessels elsewhere (NVE). New vessels leak (producing oedema and exudates), and are at risk of rupture and haemorrhage. NVF confer the greatest risk of haemorrhage. NVD indicate widespread retinal ischaemia. Proliferative retinopathy changes are pre-retinal.

4. *Advanced*. Vitreous haemorrhage, tractional detachment, rubeosis.

Any of these stages may coexist with diabetic maculopathy

Classification of diabetic maculopathy

1. *Focal*. Leakage, shown by discrete areas of HE and retinal oedema in association with ma or IRMA. Haemorrhage is variable.
2. *Diffuse*. Signs of leak diffusely throughout macula. Widespread oedema, without clear relationship between identifiable source and exudate.
3. *Ischaemic*. Closure of the macular capillary bed around the foveal avascular zone (FAZ). This can only be identified by fluorescein angiography.

Treatment

General

Vessel damage is believed to be greater if diabetic control is poor. Similarly hypertension, smoking, and lipid disorder reduce circulation and perfusion. These general risk factors must be addressed.

Ocular

Background
No treatment is indicated.

Preproliferative
Not an absolute indication for treatment, but if rapidly progressive, treatment at this stage may retard or prevent proliferation.

Proliferative
Treat by PRP using the argon or diode laser. Photocoagulation is thought to
work by ablating the retinal receptors, thereby reducing the oxygen requirement
of the retina. Elimination of ischaemic retinal mass removes the neovascular
stimulus.

Practical aspects of PRP are described in Chapter 14, p. 261. Retrobulbar
anaesthesia may be helpful, and the patient should be warned of possible visual
problems (temporary blurring, loss of field, nyctalopia, spottiness) after the treatment. Eyes with proliferative retinopathy treated by PRP have a six times lower
rate of blindness than untreated eyes with proliferative diabetic retinopathy.

Advanced
Continuing fibrovascular proliferation leads to membrane formation, vitreous
haemorrhage, and traction retinal detachment. Management of these complications requires consideration of vitrectomy surgery, which may be necessary to
flatten a macula elevated by contracting membranes, to stabilize an unstable
retina, or to remove vitreous haemorrhage.

Rubeosis usually leads sooner or later to absolute glaucoma, and a painful
blind eye. It sometimes regresses following extensive heavy PRP. Rubeotic
glaucoma can sometimes be controlled by tube and plate drainage surgery, or
may be treated by cyclocryotherapy. Alternatively, painful blind eyes may be
managed symptomatically, using topical steroid and atropine, retrobulbar
neurolytic injection, or enucleation.

Diabetic maculopathy
In focal and diffuse diabetic maculopathy the macula is damaged by accumulation of fluid and lipoprotein within the retina, caused by capillary leakage; in
ischaemic maculopathy the damage is caused by closure of the capillaries
supplying the macula (demonstrated by fluorescein angiography). Treatment
depends on an understanding of the processes threatening sight in each case.

'Clinically significant maculopathy' is defined according to macular thickening, which is caused by oedema:

● thickening within 0.5 mm of the centre
● hard exudate within 0.5 mm of the centre associated with thickening
● thickening >1 disc diameter, any part of which is within 1 disc diameter of
  the centre

Treatment is directed at closure of the leaking points, using argon green or
dye laser at 577 nm, 100 μm spot-size, 0.1 s, of sufficient intensity to whiten the
vessel or microaneurysm. Pretreatment with a lighter larger spot to produce
whitening permits closure of ma with higher power focal burns. Leaking points
are identified by the relation of ma and vessel abnormalities to HE and oedema,
or by fluorescein angiography. The treatment of diabetic maculopathy is described
in Chapter 14, p. 262.

Macular treatment preserves, and sometimes improves, visual acuity in focal maculopathy, has less certain benefit in diffuse maculopathy, and has no place in ischaemic maculopathy. Complications of macular treatment can include foveal burns, which must be avoided. Bruch's membrane can be penetrated, with subsequent SRNVM formation, if small high power burns are used.

Chronic ocular ischaemia and venous stasis retinopathy

Chronic retinal ischaemia, caused by reduced flow due to carotid or aortic arch stenosis, or hyperviscosity states (polycythaemia, leukaemia), produces a clinical picture which resembles diabetic retinopathy. CWS and retinal neovascularization indicate generalized ischaemia. The underlying vascular or haematological disease should be managed, and neovascularization treated by PRP.

Eales' disease

Eales' disease is a retinal vascular inflammatory disorder which usually occurs in young men under 40 years old. Retinal periphlebitis, which begins in peripheral vessels but may progressively involve more proximal segments, leads to capillary bed closure, neovascularization, and vitreous haemorrhage.

Affected retinal veins are dilated, with irregular calibre and periphlebitic inflammatory cuffs; there are retinal haemorrhages and CWS in affected retina, which resembles diabetic retinopathy. This stage may regress, or progress to cause retinal vein obstruction. Vitreous haemorrhage, which is characteristic of Eales' disease, is due to rupture of neovascular fronds through the internal limiting membrane. Fluorescein angiography shows capillary leakage and areas of shutdown, leakage from affected veins, and staining of their walls as they traverse ischaemic retina.

Pigmented fundus abnormalities

RPE and choroid contain melanin, and are normally pigmented to a variable degree. Choroidal vessels are visible beneath RPE in lightly pigmented eyes, of which albinism is an extreme example, and in myopia, when RPE is thin. Pigment abnormalities of RPE (clumping and depigmentation) are well-defined, whereas pigmented choroidal lesions have diffuse edges because they are beneath RPE. Fluorescein angiography helps define the location and nature of pigmented lesions, by demonstrating their relationship to RPE and choroid, and retinal and choroidal circulation.

Isolated pigmented areas

Choroidal naevus

A flat area of variable pigmentation with smooth edges, occurring at any age and in any part of the fundus. Overlying retinal vessels are normal and there may be drusen over the surface of the naevus. Naevi do not increase in size with time. Fluorescein angiography shows relative masking of choroidal circulation. A lesion thought to be a naevus should be photographed for later comparison, and managed by observation.

Malignant melanoma

Presentation

A raised area of variable size, location, outline, and pigmentation, which does not transilluminate. Melanin pigmentation is variable and may be absent, but there is usually patchy overlying orange pigment (lipofuscin) deposition.

Overlying retinal vessels are normal except in advanced cases which have broken through Bruch's membrane ('buttonholed') to become endophytic. There is often overlying serous elevation of the retina. There may be cells in the anterior chamber or the vitreous, simulating uveitis.

Differential diagnosis

Choroidal melanoma must be distinguished from naevus, subretinal haemorrhage, choroidal haemangioma, choroidal effusion, and metastatic tumour.

Fluorescein angiography shows blockage of the normal choroidal circulation, and sometimes an independent tumour circulation. Ultrasound is the most reliable diagnostic test. Vector A scan is used to measure tumour thickness, which is useful in demonstrating growth, and shows characteristic linear attenuation of echo by the tumour. Other investigations include chest X-ray, and liver scan and biochemistry, to exclude metastasis.

A staff opinion to discuss management of melanoma is arranged in most units.

Treatment

Small anterior tumours may be treated by local resection, and small and medium sized posterior tumours (<2 disc diameters), in eyes with good visual function, are increasingly being treated conservatively, with radioactive plaques, or proton beam radiotherapy.

Larger tumours, and those in eyes with poor visual prognosis, are treated by enucleation. It has been suggested that preoperative radiotherapy may reduce the incidence of recurrence following enucleation.

A small slow-growing tumour in elderly patients with good vision, or a tumour in an only eye, may be managed conservatively.

Prognosis depends principally on the cell-type of the tumour, which determines its rate of growth and metastasis. Anaplastic and epithelioid tumours have the worst prognosis, and spindle cell tumours are least aggressive.

RPE hypertrophy

Single discrete flat plaques of dense black pigmentation with irregular outline, and normal overlying retina and vessels. Visual function is not affected, the lesion is non-progressive, and intervention is not indicated.

Chorioretinal scars

Inflammation of the retina and choroid, due to physical, infective, or inflammatory causes, results in a chorioretinal scar with pigment clumped around the edges of a central atrophic area. Scars are flat, with a ragged irregular outline, and are often multiple.

Toxoplasma retinochoroiditis

The commonest infective cause of retinochoroiditis is *Toxoplasma gondii*, in which recurrences produce renewed inflammation and scarring at the edges of old lesions, and as 'satellites', separated from inactive scars. Active inflammation is indicated by blurred raised pale edges, with cells in the overlying vitreous. Antibodies are commonly positive without active inflammation. Diagnosis of toxoplasmosis is made on clinical grounds; although a rising antibody titre indicates activity, serology offers little practical help in clinical management (except inasmuch as negative serology excludes *Toxoplasma*).

Toxoplasma retinochoroiditis is treated actively if the macula, papillomacular bundle or optic disc is threatened, using prednisolone with or without antimicrobial therapy (clindamycin or pyrimethamine and a sulphonamide). Treatment is not indicated for peripheral lesions. Antimicrobial therapy has not been shown with certainty to reduce morbidity, and may be complicated by side-effects.

Subretinal haemorrhage

Subretinal haemorrhage usually occurs at the posterior pole as part of the evolution of disciform macular degeneration, as a dark submacular mass with a smooth outline. It is caused by bleeding from the SRNVM, and usually progresses to scarring, though the haemorrhage may break through the retina to enter the retrohyaloid space or the vitreous. The other eye often shows degenerative macular changes, particularly drusen. Loss of central vision occurs fairly rapidly (though it may not have been noticed). Fluorescein angiography shows masking of choroidal fluorescence.

Choroidal effusion

Choroidal effusion occurs in eyes with low pressure, usually following drainage surgery, but sometimes in association with retinal detachment. There is a smooth-contoured, globular, dark elevation of peripheral choroid and ciliary body, of which the anterior (peripheral) border cannot be identified. Choroidal effusions are usually inferotemporal and often multiple, sometimes extending deeply into the vitreous cavity.

The effusion generally resorbs as hypotony resolves. Test for wound leak, and pad the eye for 24 h if the leak is small, or resuture if it is large or the wound gapes. Dilate intensively and give topical steroid; oral acetazolamide may sometimes accelerate resolution. Surgical drainage of the effusion through the pars plana, and reformation of the anterior chamber with air via a surgical cyclodialysis, may be necessary if the effusion persists longer than a week in the presence of a flat anterior chamber.

Melanocytoma

Melanocytoma is an unusual dense black lesion, usually adjacent to disc, which occurs exclusively in dark-skinned races. It is not malignant.

Diffuse and scattered pigmented fundus abnormalities

Retinitis pigmentosa (RP)

The term 'retinitis pigmentosa' refers to a group of hereditary retinal degenerations, which involve rods initially, and ultimately all receptors, in both eyes. Inheritance may be dominant, recessive, sex-linked or sporadic. Visual loss is greater and occurs earlier in sex-linked and recessive RP, but the clinical picture is very variable.

Clinical features

RP generally presents with nyctalopia (night blindness), gradually reducing acuity and constricting field. There may be profound visual disability despite good acuity, because of severe field constriction. Visual function worsens progressively with age.

Signs

1. Perivascular retinal pigmentation scattered over the equatorial fundus in clumps resembling 'bone spicules', and progressing towards the posterior pole. Atypical forms occur, with sectoral involvement, little pigmentation, or early central involvement.
2. Retinal vessel attenuation. These vessels become extremely thin in advanced RP.
3. Waxy pallor of the optic disc.
4. Cataract, which is typically posterior subcapsular, but may take any form.

Electrodiagnosis

Electro-oculography (EOG) impairment (reduced or absent light rise) occurs early, often preceding clinical signs.

Electroretinography (ERG) shows reduced amplitude a-wave (scotopic). Photopic responses are affected later.

Variants and RP associated with systemic disorder

Pigmentary retinopathy, including early loss of photopic ERG, is part of many rare inherited diseases, of which some have a metabolic component. These include:

1. *Leber's amaurosis*. A form of RP which presents with poor vision or blindness in infancy, associated with nystagmus and an extinguished ERG. It is recessively inherited, and ophthalmoscopic signs of pigment disorder are delayed.

2. *Usher's syndrome*. Pigmentary retinopathy with sensorineural deafness.
3. *Kearns Sayre disease*. RP with cardiac conduction defects, including heart block.
4. *Refsum's syndrome*. RP with polyneuritis and cerebellar ataxia, due to phytanic acid storage disorder.
5. *Abetalipoproteinaemia*. RP with polymyopathy and progressive CNS degeneration. Haematological investigation shows crenellated erythrocytes.

Treatment of RP

No treatment is available which alters the course of RP. However, the best may be made of such visual function as remains by correcting ametropia, providing low vision aids, and encouraging support services to provide suitable educational arrangements. Cataract may contribute considerably to visual impairment, and cataract extraction with intraocular lens may be very helpful. Genetic counselling should be offered to those in whom a hereditary pattern can be established.

Other pigmentary retinopathies

Abnormal peripheral retinal pigmentation, without the other signs of RP, occurs in:

- Trauma
- Inflammation   syphilis, rubella, measles.
- Drug-induced   phenothiazines and chloroquine.
- Reattached retinal detachment
- PRP   diffusely scattered irregular fundus pigmentation. Disc pallor follows extensive heavy PRP.

Cone–rod degeneration

Some unusual tapetoretinal degenerations involve cones preferentially. In cone–rod dystrophy there is a photophobia and reduced visual acuity, with abnormal macular pigmentation which often develops into a bull's-eye maculopathy. ERG shows selective loss of photopic and flicker response.

Non-pigmented fundus abnormalities

Fundus flavimaculatus

Fundus flavimaculatus and Stargardt's disease are related disorders characterized by yellow subretinal flecks and a 'beaten bronze' macular appearance. They are recessively inherited, and present with progressive visual loss beginning during childhood, adolescence, or in young adults. Initially there are no definite ophthalmological signs, and electrodiagnosis is normal, but the visual acuity decreases to about 6/60, as the macula takes on a metallic brown sheen, with granular pigmentation and a window defect on fluorescein angiography. The extramacular retina develops yellow flecks described as 'pisciform' (fish-shaped), which initially mask choroidal fluorescence on fluorescein angiography, and later transmit it through focal atrophic RPE window defects.

Retinoblastoma

Retinoblastoma presents exclusively in infants under the age of 4 years, and is more fully considered in Chapter 10, p. 209. Dense fibrotic scars on the retina indicating treated or regressed retinoblastoma are occasionally seen in older patients.

Toxocara

Toxocara canis is a nematode parasite of dogs, which infects children who ingest the ova from ground contaminated by infected dog faeces. Larvae hatch and migrate through the body, sometimes lodging in the eye, where they may settle in any tissue. Granulomatous inflammation associated with uveitis surrounds the worm. A granuloma in the fundus presents with a large white inflammatory and fibrotic mass, which can destroy vision. Treatment is with thiabendazole and oral steroids.

Other extramacular abnormalities

Myopic degeneration

Myopic degeneration refers to areas of the myopic fundus in which retina or RPE, or both, are deficient, revealing choroidal vessels or bare sclera. Visual acuity is impaired if the macula is involved, or if Bruch's membrane beneath the macula is penetrated by subretinal neovascularization (Foster–Fuchs' spot).

Tears in the pre-equatorial retina, leading to rhegmatogenous retinal detachment, may occur as the posterior vitreous separates from the retina. Posterior staphyloma is an ectatic 'aneurysm' of the posterior pole, usually including the disc, seen in highly myopic eyes.

Choroidal folds

Choroidal folds are radial or circumferential corrugations of the choroid and retina at the posterior pole. They may be idiopathic, or secondary to a retrobulbar or choroidal mass, or thyroid ophthalmopathy. Fluorescein angiography shows alternate hypofluorescent and hyperfluorescent lines.

Angioid streaks

Angioid streaks appear as crazed lines across the fundus which appear to radiate from the disc, and are crossed by normal retinal vessels. They occur in pseudoxanthoma elasticum, Ehlers–Danlos syndrome, Paget's disease, and acromegaly, and are sometimes idiopathic. Angioid streaks represent defects in Bruch's membrane and RPE, and predispose to SRNVM. The streaks show as hyperfluorescent window defects, without leakage, on fluorescein angiography.

Choroidal haemangioma

Choroidal haemangioma is common in Sturge–Weber syndrome (multiple haemangiomas in unilateral trigeminal distribution), but may occur as an isolated abnormality.

Signs

Regular retinal elevation at the posterior pole, with mottled depigmentation of overlying RPE, and serous elevation of neuroretina.

Fluorescein angiography shows rich circulation simultaneous with choroidal filling, fluorescing throughout the arterial and venous phases. Ultrasound examination shows many highly echogenic foci within the haemangioma.

4(b) MACULA

Clinically, the macula appears as a featureless area between the temporal vessel arcades. It is centred 1.5 disc diameters temporal to the disc, and covers an area of some 2 disc diameters. At its centre is the fovea, a small reflective dimple.

Histologically, the macula is that part of the retina whose ganglion cell layer is more than one cell thick, with an abundance of cones in the photoreceptor layer; the fovea has cones exclusively, no ganglion cells, and is contained within the 200 μm radius FAZ. These anatomical arrangements give the fovea its high visual performance, but also make it particularly vulnerable to ischaemic, exudative, inflammatory, and metabolic damage.

Macular lesions which present in older individuals are usually degenerative, while those presenting below the age of 40 years are often hereditary. The principal symptom of macular disease is decreased visual acuity, with sparing of peripheral (navigational) vision and normal pupil reflexes. There may also be distortion (metamorphopsia), and reduced or altered colour vision.

Examination

Adequate examination of the macula requires dilated pupils (after testing for RAPD).

Indirect ophthalmoscope

It is useful to begin every examination of the posterior segment with the indirect ophthalmoscope, in order to gain an overall view of the backs of both eyes, including the retinal vasculature, and to compare the two maculas and discs.

Biomicroscopy

Examine the macula in detail at the slit-lamp, using the 90D or 78D lens, or a fundus contact lens such as the *area centralis*. This examination gives a high-quality stereoscopic view, revealing thickening, cystic intraretinal pathology, elevation due to subretinal fluid or haemorrhage, and pre-macular membranes. The binocular view obtained at the slit-lamp is superior to the direct ophthalmoscope's monocular view.

Fluorescein angiography

Abnormalities in the macular pigment epithelium show as window defects, revealing underlying choroidal fluorescence. SRNVMs hyperfluoresce in a characteristic 'lacey' pattern, and light up earlier than the surrounding macula, which is perfused by the retinal circulation. Cystoid macular oedema (CMO) shows as gradually increasing diffuse staining, sometimes taking a 'petalloid' pattern. Serous macular elevation due to central serous retinopathy shows a smooth-outlined, regular area of hyperfluorescence, beginning at a focus, and gradually increasing in area and intensity. Areas of haemorrhage, whether intraretinal or subretinal, mask underlying choroidal fluorescence, and appear dark. Macular drusen hyperfluoresce, creating a pigment epithelium 'window defect' through which underlying choroidal fluorescence is unmasked.

Acquired maculopathy

Cystoid macular oedema (CME or CMO)

Symptoms and signs

CMO causes reduced visual acuity, to an extent which depends on its severity and duration. Biomicroscopy shows thickening of the macular retina, with intraretinal cystic spaces, and fluorescein angiography shows persistent staining of the macula in a 'petalloid' pattern, with irregular and poorly defined edges, after the retinal veins have emptied.

Aetiology

1. *Vascular*: retinal vein occlusion (macular, temporal branch, or central); microvascular occlusion and leak in diabetic retinopathy.
2. *Inflammatory*. Complication of: uveitis (especially intermediate and posterior); posterior scleritis; retinal vasculitis.
3. *Iatrogenic*: surgical vitreous loss; PRP; side-effect of topical adrenalin therapy in aphakic eyes.
4. *Hypotony*.

Clinical course and treatment

Spontaneous resolution may occur in inflammatory cases, when vascular permeability is reduced by controlling inflammation; indomethacin or retrobulbar steroid injection may help. CMO due to vascular occlusion resolves spontaneously only if collateral channels bypass the occlusion. Focal and grid laser treatment are effective in some cases of diabetic macular oedema. Macular hole may follow chronic CMO, as the cystic spaces coalesce and rupture through the surface.

Central serous retinopathy (CSR)

Smooth localized elevation of the macular retina, caused by idiopathic leakage of choroidal extravascular fluid through a focal RPE defect. CSR typically affects young adults.

Symptoms

Blurred vision (6/12–6/36), metamorphopsia or micropsia, or a 'dark hole' in central vision. The vision often improves with a + 1D lens, because macular elevation makes the eye relatively hypermetropic.

Signs

Smooth, round, shallow elevation of the macula, best seen on biomicroscopy.

Fluorescein angiography shows an early central hyperfluorescent focus, from which a plume, or 'smokestack' of dye progressively fills the subretinal space in the area of the CSR, elevating the macula. This hyperfluorescent central area has a smooth round border which merges gradually into adjacent non-fluorescing normal retina. It persists after retinal vessel emptying, without enlarging in size.

Treatment and clinical course

CSR resolves spontaneously in 2–12 months, but recurrences are not uncommon. Focal laser treatment to close the RPE defect may shorten the duration of the serous detachment and visual symptoms, but does not significantly affect the final visual outcome or rate of recurrence.

Cellophane maculopathy (epiretinal membrane, macular pucker)

Fibroglial proliferation at the vitreoretinal interface leads to epiretinal membrane (ERM) formation, and contraction of the ERM leads to macular pucker, producing symptoms of metamorphopsia and reduced acuity. The proliferative response may follow proliferative diabetic retinopathy, retinal detachment, detachment surgery, or inflammatory or exudative maculopathy (secondary to posterior segment inflammation). The pucker is most easily seen as retinal vessel tortuosity around the macula. Reduced visual acuity in cellophane maculopathy is caused by the optical effect of the membrane on the macular image, together with macular damage (e.g. CMO) caused by the underlying pathology. ERMs can be peeled from the macula using microsurgical vitrectomy techniques.

Pigment epithelial detachment (PED)

PED presents as a dome-shaped smooth elevation of the RPE associated with reduced acuity, occurring spontaneously after middle age.

Symptoms

Moderately reduced visual acuity and distortion.

Signs

A well-defined dark yellowish elevation of the RPE, best seen on slit-lamp examination with 78D lens. There is often an overlying serous detachment of the sensory retina.

Fluorescein angiography shows early, even hyperfluorescence of a smooth circular area with well-defined edges, which persists late. PED is often associated with subretinal neovascularization.

Clinical course and treatment

The majority of PEDs resolve spontaneously without treatment, unless there is subretinal neovascularization or a pigment epithelial tear. Laser treatment may accelerate resolution, but does not improve, and may worsen, the visual prognosis. The PED may fail to resolve completely if there is a SRNVM, which may bleed, and lead to a disciform macular scar. Laser treatment to close extrafoveal subretinal neovascularization may help to avoid this complication, but in other cases PED is generally managed conservatively.

Degenerative maculopathy

Senile macular degeneration

Most maculopathy occurring in older patients is degenerative, and is termed senile, or age-related macular degeneration (SMD, ARMD). Clinically, it is described as dry or wet, according to the presence or absence of serous macular detachment, caused by leakage from associated subretinal neovascularization. Either type causes loss of central vision, while peripheral (navigational) vision is preserved. In addition patients with wet SMD may complain of distortion early in the course of its evolution, caused by the serous detachment of the macular neuroretina.

No specific therapy will arrest or reverse the changes in the majority of eyes with SMD. It is, however, important to help the patient by provision of low vision aids, reassurance that the visual loss will remain confined to the central area and not spread to threaten navigational vision (and therefore independence), and to arrange partial-sighted registration if appropriate.

Dry SMD

The ophthalmoscopic appearance is variable, including drusen, and widespread pigment epithelial atrophy of the macula with irregular pigment loss or clumping. The neurosensory layer is flat, dry, and not thickened. The cause is not clear; probably degeneration occurs in the central RPE, sensory macula, Bruch's membrane and choriocapillaris, or a combination of these layers. No treatment is available to alter the course of dry SMD.

Wet SMD

The macula is elevated by sub- and intraretinal fluid, leaking from an SRNVM arising from the choroidal circulation, which penetrates defects in Bruch's membrane and the RPE. Macular elevation, oedema and serous detachment may be accompanied by subretinal haemorrhage (deep and dark), and deep hard exudates in and around the macula. SRNVM is often associated with macular drusen, but the majority of patients with macular drusen do not develop SRNVM.

Fluorescein angiography shows a lacey net of early fluorescence, later obscured by extravasated fluorescein. Retained oedema fluid causes late staining, which gradually increases in size. Subretinal haemorrhage may mask underlying choroidal fluorescence.

SRNVM is usually progressive. The evolution of the disease includes recurrent haemorrhage, fibroglial organization, and ultimately the formation of a 'disciform' scar. Sometimes haemorrhage breaks through the macula to cause retrohyaloid or vitreous haemorrhage.

SRNVM can be closed by direct laser photocoagulation. In practice only extrafoveal membranes can safely be treated in this way, in order to avoid iatrogenic foveal damage. The FAZ extends 200 μm (approximately the width of a retinal vein at the disc margin) around the foveal centre, and an extrafoveal SRNVM lies outside this zone completely, separated from the fovea by normal retina. Krypton Red, or dye at 577 nm, is used to avoid damage to adjacent receptors. Fluorescein angiography is repeated 1–2 weeks after treatment to exclude persistent leak. Closure must be complete to prevent early recurrence, but late recurrence of an apparently completely treated SRNVM is not uncommon.

Myopic macular degeneration

The myopic macula undergoes dry atrophy and subretinal neovascularization more commonly, and often at an earlier age, than SMD. Macular SRNVM in myopia may be multiple, and is often marked by a small subretinal haemorrhage (Foster–Fuchs spot).

Macular cyst, lamellar hole (pseudo-hole), and macular hole

All cause low visual acuity but good peripheral vision.

Macular holes are generally about 0.2–0.5 disc diameter in size. They may elude cursory fundus examination if they are small and shallow and the rest of the macula looks normal. They represent successive stages of degeneration of the middle and inner layers of the neurosensory retina at the fovea. The aetiology of macular cysts and holes is not clear; some may follow coalescence and rupture of cysts, while others seem to represent a structural disorder of the internal limiting membrane over the macula.

Some authorities recommend vitrectomy surgery for macular hole, though the improvement in accuity may be limited, and surgery carries significant risk of complication.

Inherited maculopathy

Inherited maculopathies may occur as disorders confined to the macula alone, as part of a generalized retinal dystrophy, or as a component of a systemic metabolic disorder. These disorders affect both eyes, but involvement may be asymmetric. It is important to bear in mind the pattern of inheritance, and provide genetic counselling to all patients with inherited disorders.

Inherited disorders affecting the macula alone

Presentation is usually with progressive central visual loss during the first or second decade of life.

Stargardt's disease (autosomal recessive)

Stargardt's is the commonest hereditary maculopathy. It usually presents during childhood or adolescence, but occasionally not until adulthood. The macular signs are variable, including pigment mottling associated with irregular pale flecks and an abnormal sheen at the macular surface, the appearance described as 'beaten bronze'. Initially central visual function may be preserved in the presence of these abnormal signs, but the acuity falls by the third decade to the order of 6/60. Fluorescein angiography shows patchy hyperfluorescence due to un-masking of the choroidal circulation by the abnormal pigment epithelium. Occasionally the yellow flecks, which are deposits of lipofuscin accumulated in the RPE, extend into the extramacular retina; this variant is called fundus flavimaculatus. ERG and EOG are minimally impaired in Stargardt's and fundus flavimaculatus, but the visual evoked response (VER) amplitude is significantly reduced.

Stargardt's must be differentiated from X-linked juvenile retinoschisis, Best's, and bull's eye maculopathies.

Best's (vitelliform) degeneration (autosomal dominant)

A dominantly inherited maculopathy, with variable penetrance and a variable clinical picture. The onset is usually in childhood, but signs may first appear at any age from infancy to the fifth decade. Central vision is moderately reduced (6/9–6/36) in the presence of 'vitelliform' degeneration, which describes the egg-like macular changes which are usually bilateral, but may be asymmetric, or appear to be unilateral. These begin classically as an 'egg-yolk', containing yellow material which is probably composed of lipofuscin and macrophages, changing over time to a 'scrambled egg' as the acuity decreases, and terminating in macular scarring, which may be accompanied by subretinal neovascularization. The signs may be more dramatic than the symptoms suggest, and are seen in family members whose vision may be relatively spared.

ERG is normal, but EOG is invariably impaired (Arden ratio < 1.4), confirming the histopathological finding of a widespread RPE disorder. EOG is also abnormal in carriers (those in whom clinical signs are absent because of low penetrance), and in the clinically 'normal' eye of a 'unilateral' case.

Inherited macular disorders as part of a chorioretinal dystrophy

Widespread retinal involvement in these conditions is reflected in the impaired ERG and EOG found in all, and in the greater visual loss which they cause.

Cone–rod dystrophy, autosomal recessive (AR)

A form of tapetoretinal degeneration in which there is early loss of cone function throughout the retina, with central pigmentary degeneration and reduction in central visual function. Rod function is also reduced, causing night-blindness. The degeneration extends progressively to involve the equatorial and peripheral retina.

Progressive cone dystrophy, autosomal dominant (AD)

Progressive decrease in central vision, beginning in the first or second decade, with photophobia and failure of colour vision. There is a variable disturbance of the macular pigment epithelium, which sometimes takes the form of 'bull's eye' maculopathy. ERG shows reduced photopic and absent flicker responses.

Leber's amaurosis (AR)

Presents with poor vision and nystagmus in infancy. Initially, there may be no abnormality in the fundus, but progressively a pigmentary retinopathy develops, with optic atrophy. The ERG response is highly attenuated or absent.

X-linked congenital retinoschisis (X-linked)

Only males are affected, and all have a schitic retinal cleavage at the macula, which may extend into the equatorial and peripheral retina. There may be associated retinal perivascular sheathing and vitreous veils. The disorder may present with vitreous haemorrhage, as the schisis involves a retinal blood vessel. ERG shows reduced or absent b-wave.

Systemic disorders with macular involvement

Cherry-red spot syndromes

Rare metabolic storage diseases in which there is abnormal lipid deposition in the retina. Gangliosidoses (Tay–Sachs, Sandhoff's and generalized gangliosidosis), metachromatic leukodystrophy, and Niemann–Pick disease all show a cherry-red spot at the macula, as well as other profound systemic abnormalities. Related disorders have other ocular abnormalities without cherry-red spot, such as corneal lipid deposition.

The principal value of recognizing the ophthalmological signs is the help they provide in making a diagnosis of a condition with profound systemic effects.

4(c) OPTIC DISC

Anatomy

The optic disc is the anterior (ocular) part of the optic nerve. It is 1.5 mm in diameter, and conveys the ganglion cell axons from the NFL of the neurosensory retina through the sclera to the orbital part of the optic nerve. At the edge of the disc the sclera separates into two layers. One continues beneath the disc as the lamina cribrosa, while the outer layer is reflected to join the dural coat of the optic nerve. The axon bundles are supported by a framework of glial cells, and pass through perforations in the lamina cribrosa to enter the orbital part of the optic nerve.

The nerve fibres enter at the edge of the disc, forming, with glial cells, the rim around its central cup. The total area of the rim is similar in all discs (since they all convey approximately the same number of nerve fibres). The ratio of cup diameter to disc diameter therefore varies according to the size of the disc. This ratio (C/D) is sometimes used to diagnose and assess glaucoma.

The central retinal artery and vein pass through the lamina cribrosa to enter the eye, but contribute little to the blood supply of the disc. This is mainly derived from the posterior ciliary vessels, which contribute to a vascular plexus in the disc both directly and via the choroidal vessels.

Disc abnormalities

The normal optic disc has a wide range of appearances. Hypermetropic eyes have small, crowded discs in which disc tissue is heaped and pink. Myopic discs are large and pale, with thin rims, and often an adjacent temporal crescent in which retina or RPE is absent. Hypermetropic discs may appear to be pathologically elevated, and it may be difficult or impossible to assess glaucoma changes in myopic discs.

Abnormalities of the disc are of four types:

- elevation,
- cupping,
- pallor,
- congenital.

Disc elevation

The disc tissue is elevated above the plane of the retina in:

- papilloedema,
- papillitis,

- vascular neuropathy,
- infiltrative neuropathy and tumour,
- hypotony,
- pseudopapilloedema—non-pathological disc elevation.

The cause of disc elevation is diagnosed by reference to its clinical features, RAPD, visual acuity and visual field. In addition, fluorescein angiography may be necessary to distinguish papilloedema from other causes of disc elevation.

Papilloedema
Disc engorgement and elevation in the presence of raised CSF pressure.

Signs
- blurred disc margin,
- hyperaemia of disc tissue,
- dilated disc capillaries,
- obliteration of disc cup and elevation of disc surface,
- NFL oedema,
- NFL haemorrhages and CWS confined to peripapillary retina,
- absent spontaneous venous pulsation at disc.

Visual fields show enlarged blind spot. *Visual acuity* is unaffected, except by transient obscurations of vision (sudden painless visual loss lasting up to 1 min with full recovery).

Fluorescein angiography shows dilated disc vessels filling with the choroidal circulation, which leak intensely, and late staining of the disc and peripapillary retina.

Unilateral papilloedema is caused by optic nerve compression by tumour or posterior orbit inflammation, and is sometimes termed disc oedema. It represents the same pathological process as papilloedema caused by raised intracranial pressure (ICP). There is tissue oedema, cloudy swelling of cells, axon swelling with accumulation of mitochondria and capillary dilatation. Papilloedema does not occur in atrophic discs. Papilloedema of one disc in the presence of optic atrophy in the other, caused by a tumour (e.g. olfactory meningioma) which has destroyed one optic nerve before obstructing CSF flow and raising ICP, is called the Foster–Kennedy syndrome. Pseudo-Foster–Kennedy describes the same signs in a patient whose unilateral optic atrophy occurred before, and independently of, the tumour. Increasing papilloedema may ultimately compromise vision if the field loss extends to involve central fixation. Vision is also affected if intracranial pathology affects the posterior visual pathway.

- raised ICP   intracranial mass: especially of posterior fossa; pituitary tumour
                     rarely causes raised ICP
                  meningitis, intracranial abscess
                  aqueduct tumour or stenosis
                  trauma
                  benign intracranial hypertension (BICH)

- local optic nerve compression   optic nerve tumour
  dysthyroid ophthalmopathy
  orbit tumour.

Management
Confirmation of papilloedema by fundus fluorescein angiography if necessary. Skull radiology and CT to identify intracranial space-occupying lesion (SOL) or ventricular dilatation. Neurological examination and referral.

Benign intracranial hypertension is a diagnosis of exclusion. It is sometimes successfully treated medically, by serial lumbar puncture, diuretics, and weight loss.

Progressive enlargement of the blind spot threatens central vision, and requires definitive reduction of ICP. Optic nerve sheath fenestration is effective in some cases, though control of ICP is sometimes not permanent.

Papillitis

Optic neuritis affecting the optic nerve head is called papillitis. It may be inflammatory or demyelinating.

Signs
- Disc elevation.
- Reduced visual acuity.
- Relative afferent pupil defect.
- Red desaturation (reduced red colour sensation in the affected eye).
- Disc tissue pink during acute inflammation, becoming pale and progressing to optic atrophy.
- May be inflammatory cells in vitreous overlying disc.
- Visual field shows a central or centrocaecal defect, and sensitivity decreased to red targets more than to white.
- Fluorescein angiography shows progressive leak into the disc, and late staining.
- VER shows latency > 120 ms.

Causes of papillitis and retrobulbar neuritis
- demyelination,
- following viral infection,
- adjacent chorioretinal inflammation,
- intraocular inflammation,
- toxic—tobacco/alcohol, methanol, drugs.

Management
The management of optic neuritis is described in Chapter 8, p. 148.

Vascular causes of disc swelling
Anterior ischaemic optic neuropathy (AION)
- Sudden painless loss of vision, characteristically altitudinal (headaches are often a prominent feature of giant cell arteritis).

- RAPD.
- The ischaemic disc is transiently swollen and pink, later becoming pale and atrophic.
- AION follows vessel occlusion caused by: giant cell (temporal) arteritis (GCA)
  arteriosclerosis,
  carotid atherosclerosis and embolization
  hypertension.

Giant cell arteritis

GCA is a common condition which is treatable and can cause complete blindness. It is important not to miss the diagnosis. Its prevalence increases with age, and it is unusual under the age of 60 years. Any artery of the head and neck with an internal elastic lamina may be involved, and the central retinal artery is generally spared. It causes anterior ischaemic optic neuropathy, and occasionally also ocular motor nerve palsy and anterior segment ischaemia.

Symptoms and signs:

- visual loss   sudden, profound, and sometimes complete (NPL), associated with RAPD
- pain   over the temples and scalp, and masseter on mastication ('jaw claudication')
- tenderness   over the temporal arteries, scalp or masseter
- palpation   the temporal arteries and often, but not always, hard and non-pulsating
- polymyalgia rheumatica   commonly associated with GCA, with malaise, low-grade fever and muscle pains.

Diagnosis

Erythrocyte sedimentation rate (ESR) and plasma viscosity are raised. ESR is the more useful parameter in diagnosis and monitoring treatment. It is commonly raised above 80 mm/h, but it may be normal.

Biopsy under local anaesthesia provides definitive confirmation of GCA. Histological diagnosis is very useful if side-effects of treatment occur. GCA may skip segments of arteries, and a negative biopsy does not exclude the condition. Treatment should be commenced if justified clinically, even in the absence of positive biopsy.

Treatment

Commence treatment with hydrocortisone 100 mg, i.v. stat, then order prednisolone 60–100 mg/day initially, reducing after 4 days by one-third, and thereafter at increasing intervals, using ESR as a guide. Treatment is usually continued for 1–2 years.

Disc swelling in hypertension
Signs   • disc oedema
        • haemorrhages on the disc and adjacent retina
        • cotton-wool spots and hard exudates
        • hypertensive retinopathy

Hypertensive papillopathy is probably a form of AION. It occurs in accelerated hypertension, usually with systolic pressure >200. Immediate referral to a physician is indicated.

Diabetic papillopathy
Occasionally early-onset diabetics present with disc swelling in conjunction with diabetic retinopathy. It is usually bilateral, with little visual loss and variable field defect, and resolves after a few months.

Papillophlebitis (incipient central retinal vein occlusion)
Occurs mainly in females 20–40 years. The signs are of CRVO with haemorrhages localized to the disc and peripapillary retina. There is usually little visual loss, and the condition resolves over several months.

Infiltrative papillopathy and tumour

Neoplastic tissue at the disc causes irregular pale elevation and blurring of its outline, and obscures the emerging retinal vessels. Vision is reduced progressively as the optic nerve is invaded by tumour.

The disc may be infiltrated by leukaemia, lymphoma, or metastatic tumour.

Optic nerve glioma occasionally arises from the optic nerve head. Astrocytoma is characteristic of tuberous sclerosis. The tumour is pale with an irregular surface, said to resemble a mulberry. Other features of tuberous sclerosis include a nodular dermatosis over the face called acne sebaceum, epilepsy, and mental retardation. Glioma of the optic nerve head also occurs in neurofibromatosis.

Hypotony

Hypotony is usually a transient complication of intraocular surgery. Occasionally, with reduced ciliary secretion, it is chronic, and is associated with disc swelling.

Pseudopapilloedema

Pathological disc swelling is simulated by several non-pathological anomalies, and fluorescein angiography may be necessary to establish a diagnosis.

Hypermetropic disc
The disc tissue is crowded, with no physiological cup, but it is not swollen and the vessels are normal.

Bergmeister's papilla
An embryonic remnant of the developing hyaloid system. Tissue in the centre of the optic disc obliterates the cup, extending forward into the vitreous.

Optic disc drusen
Pale yellowish irregularly shaped bodies, deep or superficial in the disc, which produce irregular elevation with scalloped margins. Sometimes associated with field loss, which may resemble glaucomatous or neurological defect, though the horizontal or vertical midline is never truly respected. Fluorescein angiography shows autofluorescence before dye injection, the vessels are not dilated, and there is no late staining of the disc.

Disc drusen are sometimes associated with the development of juxtapapillary SRNVM.

Cupping

The optic disc comprises an outer neural rim of ganglion cell axons and glia around a central cup, through which the central retinal artery and vein pass. The disc is sometimes surrounded by a rim of neuroretinal or RPE atrophy. Glaucoma produces enlargement of the cup; the superotemporal and inferotemporal quadrants are usually the most vulnerable and affected first. Advanced cupping is not difficult to recognize, but earlier stages require careful assessment, since the size of the physiological disc cup is variable. The area of the neural rim is the most constant quantity, since it conveys an approximately constant number of axons in all eyes. Estimation of disc cupping must therefore take account of the size of the cup relative to the size of the disc. This measurement (cup/disc ratio, or C/D) is most reliable in the vertical axis of the disc.

Signs of glaucomatous cupping

1. C/D > 0.6 (depending on the size of the disc).
2. Undermining of the base of the neuroretinal rim, giving the cup edge a steep slope.
3. Bayonetting (double bend) of the retinal vessels as they emerge from the centre of the optic nerve. The vessels delineate the edges of the cup.
4. Inequality in size or shape between the cups of the two discs.
5. Early cupping usually affects the upper or lower temporal quadrant first (producing an arcuate scotoma). Look carefully in this area for a notch.
6. Splinter haemorrhage (in the NFL) at or adjacent to the disc.
7. Altered reflex from the retinal NFL adjacent to the disc. Retina in which the axons have been damaged by glaucoma loses its reflective lustre. This can sometimes be seen with the ophthalmoscope using a red-free or polarizing filter.
8. Exposure of the lamina cribrosa at the base of the cup.

Assessment of glaucoma must always take into account the IOPs and visual fields as well as the appearance of the optic disc. Correlation of the disc appearance with field defects helps train the ophthalmologist to recognize early signs of glaucomatous disc damage.

Uncontrolled glaucoma is demonstrated by progressive field loss or increasing disc damage. It is sometimes useful to have discs photographed for future reference.

Disc pallor and optic atrophy (OA)

The disc tissue (glia and axons) and its ciliary vessel circulation give the healthy disc its pink colour; loss of these causes pallor.

Causes of disc pallor

1. *Retinal*: (a) RP and other retinal degenerations; (b) heavy PRP; (c) long-standing total retinal detachment; (d) extensive chorioretinal inflammation; and (f) metabolic—sphingolipidoses (Tay–Sachs and Niemann–Pick) due to abnormal deposition of lipids in ganglion cells.
2. *Disc*: (a) papillitis; (b) anterior ischaemic optic neuropathy (giant cell arteritis, or arteriosclerosis); and (c) chronic papilloedema.
3. *Neurological.* (a) demyelination; (b) tumour of nerve, chiasm or tract (meningioma, glioma); (c) intracranial tumour, especially pituitary; (d) orbit trauma, avulsing the optic nerve or its blood supply; and (e) Paget's disease, causing intracanalicular nerve compression orbit malformation.
4. *Nutritional and toxic*: (a) vitamin B_1 and B_{12} deficiency; (b) alcohol/tobacco amblyopia; (c) methanol; (d) heavy metal poisoning; and (e) ethambutol.
5. *Hereditary*: (a) dominant OA; (b) recessive OA; and (c) Leber's OA.

    Leber's OA occurs usually in males aged 15–30 years, and has a mitochondrial inheritance. Visual loss occurs over several weeks in one eye followed later by the other, and is severe but not absolute. In the acute phase the disc is swollen, small disc vessels are dilated, and peripapillary vessels are abnormal and tortuous.

Congenital disc anomalies

Tilted disc

Abnormal insertion of the nerve into the disc, usually bilateral, often appearing as though the nerve enters from temporally or above. Makes estimation of disc cupping difficult, and can cause field defects simulating hemianopia (though not stepped at true neurological midline).

Bergmeister's papilla

Primitive hyaloid remnant. No pathological significance (except possible confusion with swollen disc). There may also be short vascular corkscrews emerging from disc (hyaloid vessel remnants).

Morning glory syndrome

Usually unilateral development dysplasia in which multiple small abnormal retinal vessels radiate from disc, without being organized into upper and lower temporal and nasal arcades. The central disc and the peripapillary retina are atrophic, and vision is poor.

Disc coloboma

Coloboma is a defect caused by defective union of the tissues either side of the embryological cleft. It may be of any size, and at any site in the lower half of the eye, from the disc to the iris. Disc coloboma is a white atrophic area which may extend into the retina. The extent of visual impairment depends on the size and exact site on the disc.

Optic nerve hypoplasia (ONH)

Congenitally hypoplastic discs are small with a 'double ring sign'. The outer ring is caused by atrophy (or agenesis) of the peripapillary retina and RPE. This must be distinguished from the edge of the true disc, which makes the inner ring. The extent of visual impairment depends on the degree of hypoplasia. ONH is associated with absence of the septum pellucidum (a thin lamina of cerebrum connecting the corpus callosum with the fornix) in septo-optic dysplasia, in which there are also endocrine abnormalities.

Optic disc pit

An eccentric pit in the temporal part of the disc. Serous detachment of the macula is common in eyes with optic disc pits.

Myelinated nerve fibres

Myelination of the optic nerve axons usually ceases at the disc. It may extend anomalously into a patch of retina, creating a glistening silvery patch of irregular outline, whose striae radiate from the disc.

4(d) VITREORETINAL DISORDERS AND RETINAL DETACHMENT

Anatomy

The neurosensory retina is related internally to the vitreous, and externally to the RPE, from which it is separated by a potential space representing the cavity of the optic vesicle (much as the pleural and other visceral spaces represent embryological cavities). Retinal detachment is caused by opening of this space, due to accumulation of fluid or traction acting on the retina.

The RPE is a single layer of non-replicating pigment cells, whose function includes the metabolic support of the neuroretina, particularly the outer segments of the receptors. It is separated from the choroid externally by Bruch's membrane, a fibrous and elastic sheet including the basement membranes of RPE and choroid. Retinal function is impaired if the normal close relation of the neurosensory receptor layer to the RPE is disrupted by retinal detachment.

The vitreous comprises a gel of hyaluronic acid, through which passes a scaffold of collagen fibrils. Its stability is determined by the relation between its component collagen fibrils and hyaluronate molecules, and its attachment to the inner surface of the retina at the internal limiting membrane (ILM). While the healthy young vitreous is attached to the entire inner surface of the retina, with particularly dense attachment around the ora serrata (the vitreous base), changes in gel structure and at the vitreoretinal interface with age, in myopic eyes, and in certain pathological conditions, may lead to separation of vitreous cortex from retina behind the equator, and a posterior vitreous detachment (PVD). In some eyes PVD is associated with the formation of retinal breaks, through which subhyaloid fluid passes to cause a rhegmatogenous retinal detachment.

Physiology

Retinal function depends on maintenance of normal contact between the outer surface of the neurosensory retina and the inner surface of RPE. This is lost in the area of a retinal detachment, where the two tissues are separated by fluid recruited into the subretinal space from the preretinal compartment through a retinal break. Spontaneous resorption of subretinal fluid, which occurs after a retinal break has been closed surgically, suggests that RPE cells are able to pump fluid from the subretinal space into the choroid.

If a retinal break remains unclosed (often following unsuccessful surgery), RPE cells pass through it into the preretinal compartment. Here they proliferate, assuming myofibroblast-like behaviour (synthesizing collagen and exhibiting contractility); they also probably induce the transformation and proliferation of other cells (macrophages, fibroblasts, and astrocytes), directly, or mediated by growth factors and fibronectin. The end result of these processes is the formation of fibrocellular membranes in the disorder called proliferative vitreoretinopathy (PVR).

A related proliferogenic process leads to the synthesis of fibrovascular membranes seen in advanced diabetic retinopathy; in this case, however, the stimulus is not related to RPE cells which have passed through a retinal break, but probably to retinal ischaemia.

Symptoms

Symptoms of vitreoretinal disorder are caused by optical imperfections in the vitreous (floaters), vitreous stimulation of the retina due to abnormal mobility of either structure (photopsia, or 'flashers'), elevation of retinal receptors from RPE (visual field or acuity loss), or macular distortion (metamorphopsia).

Floaters

Opacities which case a shadow on the retina cause floaters. These move with the vitreous, and they therefore have a slightly sloppy relationship with fixation as the eyes move.

Causes of floaters

Hyaloid canal remnants
Common, with no pathological significance; noticed at any age, usually against a plain light surface such as a sheet of paper or the sky.

Haemorrhage
Bleeding from a retinal tear or a neovascular frond causes a shower of new floaters. Extensive vitreous haemorrhage can prevent ophthalmoscopic examination of the fundus. Retinal detachment must then be suspected if projection of a bright focal light from the four quadrants is defective or if there is a relative afferent pupil defect, and can be confirmed or excluded by B-mode ultrasound examination.

Retinal tear is the commonest cause of vitreous haemorrhage in the non-diabetic eye.

Neovascular causes of vitreous haemorrhage are diabetic retinopathy, branch retinal vein occlusion, and breakthrough from a subretinal neovascular bleed.

Operculum
A piece of peripheral retina, torn off during PVD and elevated, leaving a retinal break. The operculum can be seen with the indirect ophthalmoscope, and helps identify and locate the break.

There is a high risk of retinal detachment, and such breaks require prophylactic treatment with cryo or photocoagulation.

Posterior segment inflammation and intermediate uveitis
Posterior segment inflammation (intermediate and posterior uveitis) produces cells and exudate in the vitreous, as well as CMO. The floaters and inflammatory signs reduce when the inflammation is controlled with systemic steroid. Intermediate uveitis is sometimes complicated by peripheral neovascularization.

Photopsia

Photopsia (flashing lights) is caused by mechanical stimulation of the retina by the detached vitreous, which has become mobile within the retrohyaloid fluid; it occurs at the time of PVD (during which process a retinal break may have occurred), and for a few weeks thereafter.

Photopsia due to PVD is perceived as a momentary streak, arcing across the temporal visual field, and is normally only noticed on eye movement, in dim illumination. This must be distinguished from the visual symptoms of ophthalmic migraine, which are formed (often geometric, zig-zag, or resembling fortifications), sustained for several minutes, central, and usually binocular.

Visual loss

Field loss

Field loss which is commonly described as 'like a curtain' obscuring part of the field of one eye, advancing from the periphery towards the centre, indicates retinal detachment. The affected field corresponds with the area of detached retina (superotemporal retinal detachment gives rise to a shadow in the infero-nasal field).

Loss of acuity

Central vision is lost when the macula becomes involved in retinal detachment. Once this has occurred, central vision is often not regained fully even after the retina has been successfully reattached surgically. For this reason it is important to assess the status of the macula when assessing a newly-presenting retinal detachment.

Visual distortion (metamorphopsia)

Monocular visual distortion indicates macular surface irregularity, due to elevation or pucker. This may be caused by epiretinal membranes in diabetic maculopathy or PVR, or to serous elevation (pigment epithelial detachment, SRNVM, central serous chorioretinopathy). Macular pucker caused by epiretinal membranes can sometimes be relieved by surgical membrane-peeling.

Retinal detachment

Elevation of the neurosensory retina, separating it from the RPE, is called retinal detachment. Retinal detachment may be rhegmatogenous, tractional, or exudative.

Examination

1. Test for RAPD. This is positive in the presence of a large detachment.
2. Slit-lamp examination. (a) Exclude anterior segment pathology; (b) cells (pigment cells or red blood cells) in the vitreous are often present in retinal detachment; and (c) IOP may be reduced in retinal detachment.
3. Dilated fundus examination of both eyes. (a) *Indirect ophthalmoscope*: with the patient supine, map the detachment and identify retinal breaks. Use the 20D lens, supplemented by the 28D to gain a wider field, and indentation to improve the view of the periphery.
   (b) *Slit-lamp biomicroscopy with 78 or 90D lens*: determine whether the macula is involved in the detachment, and whether there is a macular hole. Assess whether the vitreous is attached or detached from the retina, by focusing the slit-lamp in mid-vitreous, and observing the motion of the vitreous as the patient flicks back to the primary position from looking down or to the side. PVD can be confirmed if a mobile posterior hyaloid face is identified.

Examine the fellow eye for peripheral degeneration, break or retinal detachment, and vitreous status. The predisposing features associated with retinal detachment in one eye are often present in both. New retinal breaks are unlikely to occur in eyes in which the vitreous has completely detached from the retina.

The key to managing a retinal detachment is to identify the primary break (the break which would give rise to a detachment of a given conformation if it was the only break), and all secondary breaks. A good systematic examination is that suggested by Lincoff:

1. Draw the limits of the detachment.
2. Search for the primary retinal break in the appropriate area (see section below).
3. Search for additional holes.
4. Look for signs of PVR, which may influence the surgical management of the case.
5. Assess the vitreous, using the 90D or 78D lens at the slit-lamp.
6. Examine the fellow eye for vitreous detachment, retinal breaks and retinal detachment, as well as for any other pathology. Remember that the factors which predispose to retinal detachment are commonly present in both eyes.

Lincoff described how the conformation of a retinal detachment is determined by the site of the retinal break, formulating guidelines which are followed by the great majority of detachments:

1. In superior nasal or temporal detachments, the break lies within 1½ clock hours of the higher border.
2. In total detachments, or detachments which cross the midline superiorly, the break is at 12 o'clock, or within a triangle, the apex of which is at the ora, and the sides of which intersect the equator at 1 clock hour either side of 12 o'clock.
3. In inferior detachments, the break is on the side where the fluid is higher.
4. Detachments due to inferior breaks are relatively shallow (and slowly progressive), while those caused by superior breaks are bullous (and progress quickly). When an inferior detachment is bullous, the hole lies above the horizontal meridian (and may communicate with the inferior fluid via a peripheral sinus). In these cases the contour of the detachment may vary with posture.

Rhegmatogenous retinal detachment (RRD)

Definition

A retinal detachment caused by a break in the retina, through which subhyaloid fluid passes to enter the subretinal space as subretinal fluid (SRF).

Predisposing factors

- myopia,
- posterior vitreous detachment (risk at the time of PVD),

- lattice degeneration of the retinal periphery,
- trauma—blunt or penetrating,
- retinal detachment in the other eye,
- congenital vitreoretinal abnormality (Marfan's and Stickler's syndromes).

Clinical features

The surfaces and edges of the detachment are convex. The retina is relatively mobile, unless fixed by epiretinal membranes (ERM), in PVR. A break, or breaks, in the retina can be identified clinically, usually in an area of the retina which can be predicted by the topography of the detachment (see above).

Horseshoe tears occur at the time of PVD, and are most common in myopes. Retinal detachments caused by horseshoe tears are highly elevated, and generally progress relatively rapidly. Round holes are often multiple and not associated with PVD; the detachments they produce are often bilateral, shallow, and slowly progressive. They may have pigmented lines, or 'tidemarks', indicating long-standing, or phasic progression.

A dialysis is a separation between the anterior retina and the non-pigmented epithelium of the pars plana, in the presence of normal vitreous. There are often cystic degenerative changes extending beyond the ends of the dialysis, which curves back from the ora. Detachments due to a dialysis are smooth-contoured, slowly progressive (often showing tidemarks), and are commonly bilateral, characteristically involving the inferotemporal quadrants of both eyes. So-called traumatic dialysis is associated with a 'bucket-handle' of pars plana anterior to the peripheral retinal edge, elevated by a sector of avulsed vitreous base.

Giant retinal tears (GRT) involve two or more quadrants of the retina, and are distinguished from dialyses, or very large horseshoe tears, by the presence of a detachment of the non-pigmented epithelium of the pars plana anterior to the anterior edge of the GRT. This suggests that these breaks are not caused by the same process as horseshoe tears. PVR occurs early in the natural history of detachments caused by GRT, and in particular the rolled posterior edge of the tear usually mandates vitrectomy and internal tamponade.

Eyes with congenitally abnormal vitreous (congenital megalophthalmos syndrome, Stickler's, Marfan's) are at high risk of developing retinal breaks; in these eyes the detachment progresses rapidly, and internal tamponade is usually necessary.

Management

Retinal detachment is treated by closure of the retinal break, or breaks. This can usually be achieved by external tamponade—buckling the sclera overlying the break with an explant, supplemented by cryopexy to stimulate an adhesive reaction between RPE and retina, and in most cases by trans-scleral drainage of SRF, with injection of air or gas if necessary to replace volume or provide internal tamponade. The choice of explant (silicone sponge, tyre, or encircling band), depends upon the position and distribution of the breaks. The following decisions must be made in planning the surgical management of retinal detachment:

1. Can the break be closed by a scleral buckle?
2. Is internal tamponade necessary?
3. Is the retina mobile (i.e. is membrane peeling necessary)?

Complications
Failure of retinal reattachment
The detachment will flatten providing all the breaks have been closed. If not, the retina inevitably redetatches. Redetachment is due to failure to identify a break or all breaks, imperfect closure of break(s) due to inaccurate or inappropriate buckling, inadequate cryopexy, or failure to use vitrectomy and internal tamponade in the presence of PVR.

Haemorrhage
Vitreous haemorrhage may follow sclerotomy for trans-scleral SRF drainage. The risk of this can be minimized by maintaining IOP throughout the operation.

Vitreous or retinal incarceration
Prolapse of the retina or vitreous into the sclerotomy is caused by positioning the sclerotomy over a region of flat retina or shallow detachment, or uncontrolled SRF drainage. Such incarceration carries a high risk of subsequent ERM formation and redetachment, and should be stabilized by support on a buckle, or vitrectomy.

Proliferative vitreoretinopathy
PVR is the process by which RPE cells pass through a retinal break, acquire fibroblastic and contractile capability, and give rise to ERMs. These usually occur on the surface of the retina, in regions where the vitreous remains attached, but collagen formation also occurs within the vitreous, and sometimes in the subretinal space. The effect of PVR is to stiffen and immobilize, and progressively to shorten the retina, preventing stable closure of breaks by external tamponade. As the membranes contract, traction on the retina leads to total detachment. PVR is graded clinically according to the scheme below.

Classification of PVR (Retina Society Terminology Committee):

1. Grade A. Vitreous haze and pigment cells.
2. Grade B. Vessel tortuosity, surface wrinkling, rolled posterior edge of break.
3. Grade C_{1-3}. Full thickness retinal folds, in one to three quadrants.
4. Grade D_{1-3}. Fixed folds in four quadrants: (a) D_1 open funnel; (b) D_2 narrow funnel; (c) D_3 closed funnel.

The stimulus that causes PVR is not well understood, but it is likely to involve persistence of a patent retinal break in the presence of retinal detachment, since

PVR occurs primarily in eyes with longstanding retinal detachment, especially those in which primary surgery has failed.

Surgery to reattach the retina in these eyes requires vitrectomy, supplemented by internal tamponade, using silicone oil or gas.

Tractional retinal detachment

Definition

Elevation of the retina by traction, caused by contraction of ERMs.

Causes

Fibrovascular or fibroglial epiretinal proliferation occurs in:

- advanced diabetic retinopathy,
- PVR,
- retinopathy of prematurity (ROP),
- following penetrating trauma.

Tractional forces created by ERMs may be:

a) Preretinal (Fig. 4.1)
- tangential,
- anteroposterior,
- bridging.

b) Subretinal (Fig. 4.2)

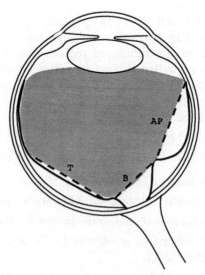

Fig. 4.1 Preretinal traction: T = tangential traction; B = bridging traction; AP = anteroposterior traction.

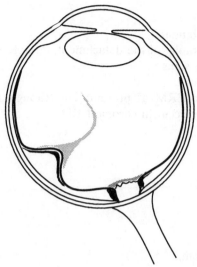

Fig. 4.2 Subretinal fibrosis. Subretinal 'washing line' and peripapillary ('napkin ring') bands.

Vision is affected in tractional detachment according to the relation of the detachment to the macula, and may remain good if the macula is spared.

The retina is shortened by the contraction of preretinal fibrous sheets or bands, and thereby elevated from the RPE. Traction detachment converts to rhegmatogenous detachment if a retinal tear develops within, or at the edge of, an area of traction.

Traction detachment may be stable, surgical intervention being indicated only if the macula is involved, or if a break develops, creating a rhegmatogenous detachment. Surgical repair is by vitrectomy and membrane peeling; internal tamponade is necessary if there are retinal breaks. Retinotomy or retinectomy may be necessary if there is severe retinal shortening, which would prevent break closure.

Exudative retinal detachment

Definition

Retinal elevation over an inflammatory, vascular, or neoplastic focus, in the absence of a retinal break or traction.

Symptoms

Visual loss, involving central vision as the macula becomes involved. Floaters and photopsia do not occur in exudative detachment. A shallow detachment is best identified using slit-lamp and 90D or fundus contact lens.

Signs
- Mobile retinal detachment.
- Shifting fluid (topography of the detachment variable with posture).
- Ocular inflammatory signs.
- Bilateral involvement.
- No retinal break or ERM at presentation (though ERM, and especially macular pucker, may occur in chronic ERD).

Aetiology

Vascular
- hypertension,
- renal disease,
- dysproteinaemia,
- SRNVM,
- Coat's disease,
- choroidal haemangioma.

Inflammatory
- posterior scleritis,
- PAN, systemic lupus erythematosus,
- sympathetic ophthalmitis,
- Crohn's disease,
- Vogt–Koyanagi–Harada syndrome.

Neoplastic
- leukaemia,
- myeloma,
- malignant melanoma,
- retinoblastoma,
- metastasis,
- orbit tumour.

Other
- central serous retinopathy,
- irradiation.

Treatment

Treat the underlying disease:

- Vascular leaks can be sealed by photocoagulation if extrafoveal.
- Inflammatory disorders are treated with systemic steroids.
- Neoplastic lesions are generally managed using radiotherapy.

Occasionally, following medical treatment of scleritis, dramatic resolution of persistent exudative detachment can be achieved by surgical de-roofing of the vortex veins.

Retinoschisis, retinal cyst

Retinoschisis results from a dissection of the retina at the level of the outer plexiform layer into an inner (inner limiting membrane, inner segments of Müller's cells, remnants of ganglion cells and nerve fibre layer, and blood vessels) and an outer (outer plexiform layer, outer nuclear layer, photoreceptors) leaf, separated by a hyaluronic acid filled cyst.

The inner leaf appears thin and transparent, light 'frosting' its diaphanous surface. Retinoschisis usually occurs in the inferotemporal quadrant, extending to the equatorial retina, and seldom involves the posterior pole; it is characteristically bilateral. Distinguish schisis from retinal detachment by the thinness of its inner leaf, which is cystic and not mobile, the absence of breaks, and the abrupt change in sensitivity at its edge on perimetry (cf. gradual loss of sensitivity across the edge of retinal detachment).

Schisis is generally stable, or very slowly progressive. Rarely it may convert into retinal detachment, if degenerative holes or tears develop in both outer and inner leaves, permitting passage of fluid from the preretinal to the subretinal space. Management is by observation; treatment is not necessary unless there is conversion to rhegmatogenous detachment.

Vitreous haemorrhage

Aetiology
1. Retinal tear, at the time of PVD.
2. Ruptured neovascular frond (diabetic retinopathy, retinal vein occlusion, occasionally intermediate uveitis or Eales' disease).
3. SRNVM bleed breakthrough (disciform macular degeneration).
4. Trauma.

Clinical features
Sudden storm of floaters, reduced acuity, reduced or abolished red reflex, poor ophthalmoscopic view of fundus. There is no relative afferent pupil defect.

Management
1. Exclude retinal detachment: (a) indirect ophthalmoscope. If view is inadequate: (b) accurate projection of light in four quadrants; (c) negative RAPD; (d) B-mode ultrasound.
2. Exclude diabetes.
3. If retinal detachment is confirmed, admit for bed rest and early vitrectomy.
4. If there is no retinal detachment, review periodically, for photocoagulation to source of retinal bleed, or PRP, when the haemorrhage has cleared sufficiently; vitrectomy is indicated if VH had not cleared after a month or two of conservative management.

Peripheral vitreoretinal degenerations

The peripheral retina extends from the equator forwards to the ora serrata. The vitreous base—the region of densest vitreoretinal attachment—is located between the pars plana and the equator. Large oral bays at the anterior insertion of the retina are developmental anomalies which may be confused with peripheral flat retinal holes; they do not predispose to retinal detachment.

Peripheral vitreoretinal degenerations are common in ageing and myopic eyes. They are bilateral, and can be classified according to the risk they carry of retinal break, and subsequent detachment.

Degenerations with low risk of retinal break

Cystoid
Multiple intraretinal cysts, especially in the temporal periphery. Peripheral cystic changes can be seen in the retina of young eyes, but become increasingly prevalent with age.

Pigmentary degeneration
Irregular pigment clumping, mottling, and focal depigmentation of the peripheral RPE is common in ageing eyes.

Cobblestone/pavingstone degeneration
Irregular, smooth-outlined pale patches, between equator and ora. The appearance of cobblestone is due to atrophy of RPE and choriocapillaris. There may be hyperpigmentation between foci. It is common, especially in ageing eyes.

Degenerations with high risk of retinal break

Lattice degeneration
Fine white lines arranged in criss-cross 'lattice' or random patterns, in association with small vessels, in pre-equatorial retina. Lattice is usually bilateral, and often located in corresponding areas in both eyes. Retinal breaks are common within or around areas of lattice degeneration, and are a common cause of retinal detachment.

Treatment with prophylactic cryotherapy is indicated if there are associated retinal breaks, or to areas of lattice in one eye in the presence of detachment in the other.

Myopic degeneration
Moderate and high myopic eyes (greater than −6D) are at particular risk of retinal break formation, and detachment. They exhibit the following features:

- early posterior vitreous detachment,
- peripapillary atrophy,
- areas of retinal atrophy, which may also involve RPE and choriocapillaris, revealing bare sclera,
- splits in Bruch's membrane ('lacquer cracks'),
- lattice degeneration,
- 'white without pressure' pre-equatorial changes,
- posterior staphyloma,
- scleromalacia,
- subretinal neovascularization through a break in Bruch's membrane (Foster–Fuchs' spot).

Retinal breaks

Horseshoe (U-shaped or arrow-head) tears

Caused at the time of posterior vitreous detachment, as focal dynamic traction forces are exerted on an area of retina in which vitreoretinal separation is incomplete. Horseshoe tears lead to rhegmatogenous retinal detachment, and require cryotherapy to create an adhesive response which will seal the break; external buckling is necessary if the break is elevated by subretinal fluid.

Round retinal holes

Round flat holes in the retinal periphery. They are present in 0.4 per cent of adult eyes, and are not associated with PVD. These holes confer a risk of retinal detachment, and are treated by prophylactic cryotherapy or photocoagulation.

Vitreous degeneration

Posterior vitreous detachment (PVD)

The tertiary structure of the vitreous changes with age, and it eventually separates from the posterior retina. This posterior vitreous detachment (PVD) is symptomatic, producing flashing streaks, usually noticed in the upper temporal quadrant in darkness, and floaters. PVD occurs at a younger age in myopes. PVD can be identified at the slit lamp by observing the free posterior hyaloid face; Weiss' ring, which is the former attachment to the disc, can often be seen in the midvitreous with the indirect opthalmoscope.

Syneresis

Cavities form within the ageing vitreous, and give rise to floaters. They may resemble a PVD on biomicroscopy, but can be distinguished by the absence of a posterior hyaloid face.

Asteroid hyalosis and synchisis scintillans

In asteroid and synchisis there are many small discrete bodies in the vitreous, which do not usually impair vision, but often reduce the clarity of the ophthalmoscopic view. They are best seen with the indirect opthalmoscope, on account of its depth of focus and low magnification. The opacities remain suspended throughout the vitreous in asteroid, but settle, until they are agitated by eye movement, in synchisis.

Asteroid is common, usually unilateral, and sometimes associated with diabetes. It is caused by calcified lipid soap particles suspended in the vitreous, of unknown aetiology. Synchisis is uncommon, caused by a suspension of cholesterol crystals in the vitreous, usually following vitreous haemorrhage.

No intervention is indicated in either condition unless, unusually, vision is significantly impaired.

Recommended further reading

Freeman, W.R. (1993). *Practical atlas of retinal disease and therapy*. Raven Press, New York.

Grey, R. (1991). *Vascular diseases of the ocular fundus*. Butterworths, London.

Kritzinger, E.E. and Beaumont, H.M. (1987). *A colour atlas of optic disc abnormalities*. Wolfe, London.

Michaels, R.G., Wilkinson, C.P., and Rice, T.A. (1990). *Retinal detachment*. Mosby, St Louis.

Ryan, S.J. (1989). *Retina*, vols I–III. Mosby, St Louis.

Yannuzzi, L.A., Gitter, K.A., and Schatz, H. (1979). *The macula. A comprehensive text and atlas*. Williams & Wilkins, Baltimore.

5

Glaucoma

Glaucoma describes a number of ocular conditions characterized by:

- raised intraocular pressure (IOP),
- optic nerve head damage,
- corresponding loss of visual field (VF).

IOP depends on the relationship between aqueous production and outflow. In practice the principal determinants of IOP are the factors which limit outflow facility. These may be structural or functional, congenital or acquired, or primary or secondary. In addition it is clear that the sensitivity of the optic nerve head to IOP varies among individuals, and in the context of established glaucoma, VF loss may be more or less dependent on the level of IOP.

Classification

The clinical picture and management depend on the underlying pathology, which is classified according to three principal parameters:

- angle   open
                 narrow/closed
- onset   acute
                 chronic
- aetiology   primary
                 secondary

Glaucoma presents most commonly as one of three clinical types:

- primary open angle glaucoma (POAG)
- acute angle closure glaucoma (AACG)
- secondary glaucoma

Sometimes elements of more than one type are superimposed (e.g. POAG may be complicated by progressive angle narrowing in the presence of an intumescent cataract, or secondary glaucoma added in the presence of anterior uveitis). There are also several glaucoma syndromes associated with specific structural and functional abnormalities, described below.

Signs

Intraocular pressure

21 mmHg represents 2 standard deviations above the mean IOP of a population of healthy eyes; eyes with IOP above this are at significantly increased risk of optic nerve damage and field loss. The IOP shows physiological diurnal variation, and can be artefactually raised during measurement, e.g. by lid pressure.

Visual field

The VF is recorded to establish the diagnosis and monitor progression and the effect of treatment. Several different techniques of VF measurement, or perimetry, are available. Computerized perimeters (e.g. Humphrey, Octopus, Dicon) are automatic, can be very accurate, but are expensive; the Henson is a simple automated perimeter, which is not difficult to use. The Goldman is sensitive, accurate, and versatile, but requires some skill to use; Friedman requires little skill, but gives limited clinical information.

Perimetry is carried out as either a kinetic (stimulus moved from periphery to centre until it is perceived) or static (intensity of a stationary stimulus increased until it is perceived) procedure. Both static and kinetic procedures can be used with the Goldman; Friedman and most automated perimeters use static procedures. The sensitivity in a normal eye varies across the field, being greatest centrally, and progressively less toward the periphery; sensitivity at the blind-spot (projection of the optic disc) is zero. The strategies employed clinically to identify the distribution of sensitivity across the field can be divided into 'threshold' and 'suprathreshold' routines; threshold perimetry quantifies the minimal perceivable stimulus at each point in the field, while suprathreshold tests identify any part of the field in which sensitivity is reduced below the expected level for that eye, in relation to reference thresholds. Suprathreshold procedures are relatively fast, and are useful for screening. Threshold tests are time-consuming, can give more information, but are often tiresome to patients, which can limit their usefulness.

Field changes in glaucoma show several characteristic patterns:

1. Arcuate scotomas arch around fixation to the blind spot, following the anatomical pattern of the retinal nerve fibres. The upper and lower temporal segments of the disc are most vulnerable to damage by glaucoma, giving rise to variable sensitivity in the arcuate areas 10°–15° above and below fixation.

2. The path of the nerve fibres is separated by a horizontal raphe passing through the macula to the disc, giving rise to a characteristic 'nasal step' in sensitivity across the horizontal midline in the nasal field, which can be demonstrated by moving a threshold target up and down over the midline in this zone.

3. In the temporal field, scotomas are characteristically wedge-shaped, due to the radial entry of nasal fibres into the optic nerve.

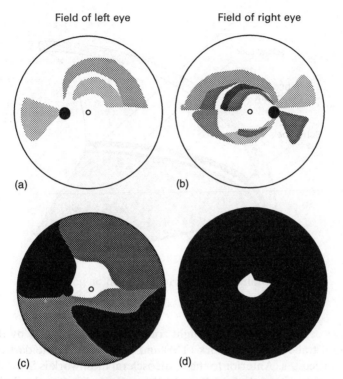

Field of left eye   Field of right eye

(a)   (b)

(c)   (d)

Fig. 5.1 Glaucoma. Progression of field loss.

Figure 5.1 shows progressive loss of field caused by glaucoma.

During an attack of acute glaucoma all visual function is reduced; following control of IOP there may be disc ischaemia, glaucomatous field loss, or complete recovery.

Optic disc (OD)

Nerve fibres (ganglion cell axons) enter the optic nerve through the neuroretinal rim of the OD, around its central physiological cup. Loss of these nerve fibres and associated glial tissue in glaucoma causes pathological cupping.

Drainage angle

The drainage angle is examined by gonioscopy, to assess its anatomy, and identify pathology. The goniolens is a small contact lens incorporating a prism, which permits an image of the angle to escape total internal reflection by the cornea, and emerge to be examined at the slit-lamp.

The features of the angle seen on gonioscopy are shown in Fig. 5.2. The scleral

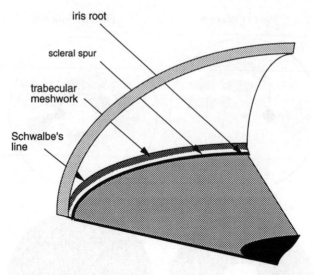

iris root

scleral spur

trabecular
meshwork

Schwalbe's
line

Fig. 5.2 Drainage angle structures seen on gonioscopy.

spur is most easily identified, as a light zone bounded anteriorly by the darker corneoscleral trabecular meshwork (TM) and posteriorly by the darker iris root and ciliary processes. Anterior to the corneoscleral meshwork is Schwalbe's line, which is variably pigmented, and marks the anterior limit of the TM, and the posterior limit of Descemet's membrane. Sampaolesi's line and posterior embryotoxon are dark lines sometimes seen anterior to Schwalbe's.

The angle is safely open if the TM and the scleral spur can be seen. Only anterior TM and Schwalbe's line can be seen in narrow angles, and if no angle structures can be seen there is a high risk of closure, which may be precipitated by pupil dilatation. The angle is always narrower temporally than nasally, and where peripheral anterior synaechiae (PAS) occur, they obliterate all angle structures.

Primary open angle glaucoma

1. *Incidence*: 0.5–2 per cent of the population over 40 years.

2. *Risk factors*: age (>40 years): positive family history; diabetes; myopia.

3. *Aetiology*: Unknown. Theories suggest: functional inadequacy of TM drainage; hypoperfusion of optic nerve head; and weakness of structural collagen in the angle and disc.

4. *Symptoms*: none until late, when considerable field loss has already occurred; not associated with pain, discomfort or redness; new cases are usually identified by screening.

Signs

Intraocular pressure

In ocular hypertension (OHT, 'glaucoma suspect'), IOP is elevated without disc or field changes. A proportion of eyes with OHT ultimately develop glaucoma. In low tension glaucoma (LTG) there are disc and field changes characteristic of glaucoma, without elevated IOP. A diagnosis of LTG should not be made unless CT scan has excluded a compressive lesion of the optic nerves or chiasm as a cause of field and disc changes; chiasm compression (most commonly by pituitary tumour) may cause field changes which do not display classical hemianopic features.

Visual fields

Up to 50 per cent of ganglion cell axons entering the disc may be lost before disc and field changes are evident. The earliest detectable field abnormalities are patches of variable sensitivity in a zone 10°–20° above or below fixation. These develop into arcuate scotomas, which approach or join the blind spot. Peripheral field is progressively lost, but central acuity is affected late.

Individual patients often show variability between successive fields, which does not reflect progressive field loss. Consistent field loss progression indicates that treatment is inadequate and should be altered.

Disc

Damage usually begins as an upper or lower temporal notch, giving rise to a nasal arcuate scotoma. The extent of cupping is assessed as the vertical cup/disc ratio, which is recorded as a fraction (C/D).

The principal features of glaucomatous cups are:

- right/left asymmetry,
- enlargement to more than 60 per cent of the vertical disc dimension (C/D > 0.6),
- undermining of the cup edge,
- bayonetting of retinal vessels passing over the disc edge,
- shift of vessels to the nasal edge of the disc,
- splinter haemorrhage at the edge of the disc.

The absolute size of the cup may be misleading, since it is the volume of the neuroretinal rim which is important, and this is much thinner in a large disc. For this reason it can be very difficult to assess glaucoma in myopic discs.

It is sometimes useful to have a suspicious disc photographed, for later comparison.

Management

Disc cupping and field loss in POAG progress at a variable rate, leading in the most severe cases to profound field constriction and ultimately blindness. The aim of management is to lower IOP sufficiently to arrest progressive VF loss. There is no clear distinction between normal, or 'safe' and elevated or damaging levels of IOP; the adequacy of control must be assessed at each examination by reference to VF, IOP, and disc appearance in comparison with previous findings. Some optic nerve heads seem to survive IOPs at levels higher than others.

Medical treatment

Medical treatment is appropriate if it stabilizes IOP at a safe level and arrests field loss, or if surgery is contraindicated.

1. b.d. topical beta-blockers (timolol, carteolol, betaxolol, metipranolol, levo-bunolol). Beta-blockers are contraindicated in patients with asthma, bradyar-rhythmia, heart block, and cardiac failure. There is no convincing evidence that beta-blockers with cardioselective or intrinsic sympathomimetic activity are significantly safer in these patients.

2. b.d. propine to supplement beta-blockade.

Surgical treatment

Trabeculectomy provides a definitive and permanent reduction of IOP to within safe limits in the majority of cases. The procedure is much less successful in aphakic and rubeotic eyes.

Indications

- clearly diagnosed POAG,
- continued field loss in spite of medical treatment,
- young patients with established POAG and marginal control on medical treatment,
- medical treatment contraindicated.

Complications

- postoperative flat anterior chamber (leak or choroidal effusion),
- cataract,
- infection: immediate or delayed,
- failure to control IOP.

Modifications

Molteno tube (a silicone tube implant draining beneath a subconjunctival plate) and similar devices are used to maintain patency of the fistula between anterior chamber and subconjunctival space where simple trabeculectomy has failed repeatedly, or is likely to fail (e.g. in rubeotic glaucoma).

Trabeculectomy is sometimes supplemented with subconjunctival injection of 5-fluorouracil in eyes at high risk of failure due to bleb fibrosis.

Cataract and glaucoma occur in the same age group and often coexist. Cataract extraction + intraocular lens implant may be undertaken at the same time as trabeculectomy.

Laser treatment

Argon laser treatment to the trabecular meshwork (argon laser trabeculoplasty) produces a modest reduction in IOP, which is maintained for >2 years in about 50 per cent of eyes. 50–100 small high energy burns (1 W × 0.1 s × 100 μm) are applied to the anterior trabecular meshwork through a goniolens. The scarring this causes is believed to open up the intertrabecular drainage channels. Though IOP is reduced, there is often an initial rise (during the acute phase of trabeculitis), and in many eyes the IOP reduction is not permanent. This is not an alternative to trabeculectomy, but an alternative means of IOP reduction in those in whom surgery presents particular problems.

New approaches to treatment of glaucoma by laser, presently not used widely, include Holmium laser trabeculotomy and trans-scleral YAG (continuous wave) laser cycloablation.

Angle closure glaucoma (ACG)

Short eyes, which are generally hypermetropic, have a narrow drainage angle, with little space between the peripheral iris and the trabecular meshwork. This narrow angle is easily obstructed: as the pupil dilates in the presence of a thickening ageing lens, increased resistance to aqueous flow through the pupil causes a relative pupil block, and forward bowing of the peripheral iris occludes the angle.

An angle at risk of closure is diagnosed when gonioscopy reveals no visible angle structure between the peripheral iris and the peripheral cornea. In established ACG, gonioscopy is not possible on account of corneal oedema (though this can sometimes be cleared temporarily using glycerol drops to dehydrate the cloudy, decompensated cornea). It is always helpful to inspect the angle in the fellow eye in AACG, since this also is likely to be narrow, confirming the diagnosis, and indicating the need for prophylactic treatment.

The anterior chamber depth and angle can be assessed informally by shining a focal beam from the side across the eye at a tangent to the corneal surface. Even illumination of both temporal and nasal iris indicates a flat iris profile and adequate anterior chamber depth. If the nasal iris is shadowed, the angle is narrow; eyes displaying this sign should only be dilated after accurate estimation of angle anatomy has been made gonioscopically.

Angle obstruction may be:

- incomplete but progressive — chronic angle closure,
- intermittent and reversible — intermittent ACG,
- complete and irreversible — acute angle closure glaucoma (AACG).

Acute angle closure glaucoma

Clinical features

1. *Visual reduction*: due to corneal oedema and posterior segment ischaemia.
2. *Raised IOP*: usually 40–70 mmHg.

3. *Coloured haloes around lights*. Due to diffraction of light through the oede-matous corneal epithelium. Indicates subacute pressure rises, and usually presages acute angle closure.
4. *Pain*: may be severe, and associated with vomiting.
5. *Ciliary injection*.
6. *Mid-dilated pupil, often oval*: due to ischaemic iris atrophy.
7. *Corneal oedema*: due to decompensation of the corneal endothelial pump, on account of high flow from aqueous into stroma.
8. *Anterior chamber cells and flare*: due to accompanying anterior uveitis.

Treatment

Immediate

The IOP must be reduced medically as quickly as possible, using:

Diuretics
Acetazolamide to reduce aqueous production:

- 500 mg, i.v. immediately
- 250–500 mg orally, t.d.s.

If intravenous acetazolamide fails to reduce the pressure to below 35, repeat once. If the pressure remains high, give an intravenous mannitol infusion (200 ml 20 per cent mannitol, i.v. over 1–2 h). Mannitol is an osmotic diuretic, and is preferable to the oral alternative, glycerol (1.5–4 ml/kg) 50 per cent solution mixed with fruit juice, which is nauseous.

Miotics
When the IOP has been reduced to below 35 mmHg, miotics may be expected to maintain transpupil flow and angle function, unless there is an irreversible element to the angle closure. Give intensive pilocarpine therapy (every 10 min for 1 h, then hourly for 6 h). Then maintain on pilocarpine 2 per cent q.d.s., both to the affected eye, and prophylactically to the fellow.

Steroid
Give topical steroid q.d.s. during the acute phase to reduce the accompanying inflammatory response, and prevent formation of PAS, which cause further angle damage.

Analgesia
Acute angle closure may be very painful; parenteral analgesia (pethidine) and antiemetics may be needed.

Definitive treatment

Once an acute attack of ACG has been controlled medically, the eye must be protected against a recurrence, by surgery or laser treatment. If the IOP remains within normal limits for several days following discontinuation of acetazolamide, there has been no significant PAS formation, and peripheral iridectomy (surgical) or iridotomy (YAG laser) is sufficient. If IOP rises on discontinuing acetazolamide, the drainage angle has been compromised and is functionally inadequate; trabeculectomy will probably be necessary.

The fellow eye should always be protected by prophylactic YAG laser iridotomy or surgical iridectomy.

Chronic angle closure glaucoma

Clinical features

Chronic ACG is usually asymptomatic, when it may be misdiagnosed as open angle glaucoma if the angle is not examined by gonioscopy; alternatively it may begin as intermittent subacute angle closure, causing pain and haloes. The anterior chamber is shallow and gonioscopy reveals a narrow angle, sometimes with PAS.

Treatment

Medical

Pilocarpine drops q.d.s. Patients should be warned of the side-effects of pilocarpine: discomfort (pupil spasm), and reduced vision, especially in dim light, caused by miosis. These usually abate after a few weeks of treatment. If pilocarpine is ineffective in controlling pressure, surgery will probably be necessary.

Laser

YAG laser iridotomy will control chronic ACG providing substantial functioning drainage angle remains.

Surgical

Trabeculectomy is necessary if laser iridotomy fails to control IOP, indicating irreversible closure of more than 180° of the angle.

Secondary glaucoma

Aetiology

Secondary obstruction of aqueous drainage occurs in the presence of an open or a closed angle, due to many causes.

Causes of secondary glaucoma:

1. Closed angle: (a) inflammation; (b) hyphaema; (c) rubeotic glaucoma; and (d) lens-induced (phakomorphic).
2. Open angle: (a) pigment dispersion; (b) pseudoexfoliation; (c) steroid therapy (topical or systemic) in 'steroid responders'; (d) vitreous haemorrhage (ghost cell glaucoma); (e) angle recession (following trauma); and (f) vascular abnormalities.

Secondary closed angle glaucoma

Inflammation

If posterior synaechiae scar 360° of the pupil to the lens, aqueous flow from the posterior to the anterior chamber is obstructed, elevating the aqueous pressure in the posterior chamber and causing iris bombé. The peripheral iris then occludes the drainage angle, and in the presence of active anterior segment inflammation the occlusion rapidly becomes irreversible on account of PAS.

Secondary glaucoma in the presence of iris bombé is treated by:

1. Intensive mydriasis to break the pupil block.
2. Intensive topical steroid to reduce the inflammatory response.
3. Surgical peripheral iridectomy, or YAG laser iridotomy, when the cornea is sufficiently clear. Satisfactory full-thickness iridotomy is indicated by a plume of pigment and blood into the anterior chamber, accompanied by immediate deepening.

Prevention of synaechia formation, to avoid the complication of secondary glaucoma, is one of the principal aims of the treatment of acute anterior uveitis.

Hyphaema

Elevated IOP may accompany total hyphaema, especially if this follows a second-ary re-bleed. The IOP rise is due to pupil obstruction by the clot, and is treated by intensive dilation. If the IOP remains high in the presence of hyphaema, the corneal endothelium may stain irreversibly with haemoglobin.

Rubeotic glaucoma

Rubeosis describes the anterior and posterior segment neovascularization which occurs in severely ischaemic eyes. It occurs in advanced proliferative diabetic retinopathy, following central retinal vein occlusion (CRVO), in chronic ocular ischaemia, and in the presence of longstanding total retinal detachment. New vessels proliferating in the anterior segment grow from the pupil towards the drainage angle, which becomes irreversibly obstructed.

Medical treatment is generally ineffective in rubeotic glaucoma, which is best managed by prevention: the retina in eyes with ischaemic CRVO and proliferative diabetic retinopathy must be treated with sufficient panretinal photocoagulation to cause regression of neovascularization. Regression of established rubeosis sometimes follows heavy panretinal photocoagulation. Trabeculectomy in rubeotic eyes is usually unsuccessful, but may be supplemented with a perma-nent silicone tube anterior chamber fistula connected to a subconjunctival plate (e.g. Molteno tube), to prevent obliteration of the surgically formed drainage pathway. Cyclocryotherapy is sometimes successful in reducing IOP, by re-ducing aqueous production.

Lens-induced glaucoma

Dislocated or subluxed lenses are frequently associated with glaucoma. This may be due to pupil block, or if the lens has dislocated into the vitreous, to chronic inflammation.

Hypermature and traumatic cataracts leak lens protein through a pathologically permeable capsule, and may give rise to secondary glaucoma.

Treat pupil block with cycloplegia and steroids. Surgical removal of a dislocated lens is hazardous, and if necessary requires lensectomy using vitrectomy instrumentation.

Secondary open angle glaucoma

Pigment dispersion

Pigmentary glaucoma is a form of open angle glaucoma occurring in conjunction with the pigment dispersion syndrome. It generally affects younger patients, causing shedding of iris pigment and transillumination defects. Pigment accumulates in the angle, where it can readily be seen gonioscopically; it also accumulates on the central zone of the corneal endothelium, as Krukenberg's spindle. Pigment dispersion may occur without glaucoma. Trabeculectomy is usually successful in controlling IOP.

Pseudoexfoliation

Flaky or fluffy white material (proteoglycan) accumulates in a ring on the anterior lens capsule and at the pupil margin. It also accumulates in the drainage angle, often together with pigment. Glaucoma occurs in up to 50 per cent of eyes with pseudoexfoliation. Pseudoexfoliation and glaucoma are usually bilateral but asymmetric.

Steroid-response glaucoma

All eyes respond to topical steroid administration with a rise in IOP. In most this is a modest rise, which occurs only after several weeks' treatment, but in about 20 per cent the rise is clinically significant; these individuals are called 'steroid responders'. There is an increased prevalence of steroid response among individuals with POAG. Steroid-induced glaucoma is a particular risk in long-term steroid use without adequate ophthalmic supervision. It may also account for some cases of postoperative high IOP immediately following trabeculectomy. IOP returns to normal when steroid use is discontinued.

Angle recession

Non-penetrating trauma may lead to disinsertion of the anterior radial fibres of the ciliary body from the scleral spur. This leads to angle recession, in which the anterior chamber looks abnormally deep, and on gonioscopy is pathologically wide, with loss of the normal architecture. Angle recession glaucoma is often delayed months or years following the trauma, and is probably caused by collapse of the trabecular meshwork.

Vascular anomalies

Elevated orbital venous pressure is transmitted through the episcleral veins to the aqueous veins draining Schlemm's canal, and causes elevation of IOP because aqueous drainage is driven by the hydrostatic gradient between intraocular and intraorbital pressure. Dilated blood-filled vessels are often visible in the angle gonioscopically.

Glaucoma of this type is seen in caroticocavernous fistula, dural shunt, and the Sturge–Weber syndrome (multiple haemangiomas distributed in the trigeminal distribution, and involving the brain).

Uveitis syndromes associated with glaucoma

As well as the mechanisms described above by which uveitis may lead to secondary glaucoma, two specific uveitis syndromes are characteristically associated with raised IOP and optic nerve damage.

Fuchs' heterochromic iridocyclitis (HIC)

A distinct anterior uveitis syndrome, characterized by crinkled keratic precipitates distributed over all the corneal endothelium (not only the inferior part), associated with atrophy of the anterior border layer of the iris, which becomes pale grey-blue and transilluminates. Posterior synaechia do not form, but cataracts and significant sustained elevation of IOP, with disc cupping and field loss, are common. Fuchs' HIC does not generally require treatment with steroid or mydriatic, but IOP needs to be controlled, with topical beta-blockers, or by trabeculectomy if medical treatment is ineffective.

Posner–Schlossman syndrome

Posner–Schlossman affects young to middle-aged adults, with recurrent episodes of mild anterior uveitis, associated with high elevations of IOP. Treatment is with topical steroids during acute attacks, supplemented if necessary with topical beta-blockers, and oral acetazolamide. Trabeculectomy is occasionally necessary.

Congenital glaucoma

Primary infantile glaucoma

Glaucoma in infants may present with pain, photophobia, watering, blepharospasm, cloudy cornea, reduced vision, or ocular enlargement. Signs include linear breaks in Descemet's membrane (Haab's striae), corneal oedema, enlarged cornea (horizontal corneal diameter > 10.5 mm at birth, > 12 mm age 1 year), raised IOP, gonioscopic angle anomalies, OD cupping. An infant with glaucoma needs periodic examination under anaesthesia in order to monitor these signs and assess the effectiveness of treatment. Most cases are sporadic, and in 75 per cent both eyes are involved.

Glaucoma associated with anterior segment cleavage anomalies

Embryological maldevelopment of the anterior segment produces a spectrum of angle abnormalities collectively called 'anterior chamber cleavage syndromes'.

Mesoderm forming the corneal endothelium, the anterior stroma of the iris and the trabecular meshwork, normally cleaves to form the anterior chamber. If cleavage is incomplete, residual mesodermal tissue obstructs access to the angle from the anterior chamber. Cleavage disorders exhibit a range of signs, from minor gonioscopic angle anomalies to serious sight-impairing abnormalities. They are associated with glaucoma, which often presents congenitally or during infancy as buphthalmos (described more fully in Chapter 10, p. 207), but whose onset may be delayed until later childhood, or adulthood. Named cleavage anomalies are usually inherited in an autosomal dominant pattern, and are categorized according to the tissues involved.

Posterior embryotoxon
A line of persistent mesodermal tissue anterior to Schwalbe's line.

Axenfeld's anomaly
Posterior embryotoxon associated with dense iris bands to Schwalbe's line. Glaucoma occurs in 50 per cent.

Rieger's anomaly
Anterior iris surface hypoplasia, dense peripheral iridocorneal bands, and posterior embryotoxon. Frequently associated with cataract. Associated dental, skeletal, and neurological disorder termed Rieger's syndrome.

Peter's anomaly
Central posterior corneal opacity with persistent iridocorneal and lens–corneal tissue bridges, and severe angle anomalies. Cataract usually occurs, and glaucoma often begins during infancy.

Treatment of congenital glaucoma
Onset of glaucoma in childhood
Early goniotomy is usually necessary to prevent visual loss. Control of glaucoma is usually difficult in severely affected eyes in spite of surgery.

Adult-onset glaucoma
Trabeculectomy is usually effective.

Aniridia
An autosomal dominant hereditary disorder of iris development in which the iris is hypoplastic or absent, and sometimes associated with foveal hypoplasia, cataract, and ectopia lentis. Glaucoma develops in late childhood or adulthood.

Malignant glaucoma

Progressive elevation of IOP with an increasingly shallow anterior chamber, following drainage surgery or cataract extraction, which is unresponsive to topical medication. Malignant glaucoma is much less common following trabeculectomy than earlier forms of drainage surgery. Normal passage of aqueous from the posterior to the anterior chamber is obstructed by the anterior hyaloid, causing pooling of aqueous behind the lens and leading to progressive forward displacement of the lens–iris diaphragm, shallowing of the anterior chamber, and secondary occlusion of the drainage angle, and raised IOP. Treatment is initially with acetazolamide to reduce aqueous formation, combined with intensive cycloplegia. If this fails it may be necessary to undertake vitrectomy, to restore normal aqueous circulation.

Absolute glaucoma

Eyes in which drainage is completely blocked develop very high pressure (50–60 mmHg), total glaucomatous cups, and corneal decompensation. Useful vision is lost, and the eye may be painful as a result of ciliary ischaemia or bullous keratopathy. The blind, painful eye is treated symptomatically:

- bandage contact lens,
- topical atropine b.d., steroid (e.g. dexamethasone) q.d.s.,
- retrobulbar neurolytic injection (phenol 6 per cent aqueous, alcohol),
- enucleation.

Recommended further reading

Cairns, J.E. (1986). *Glaucoma* (2 vols). Grune & Stratton, London.
Hoskins, H.D. (1989). *Becker & Schaffer's diagnosis and therapy of the glaucomas*, 6th edn. Mosby, St Louis.
Kanski, J.J. and MacAllister, J.A. (1986). *Glaucoma. A colour manual of diagnosis and treatment*. Butterworths, London.
McAllister, J.P. and Wilson, R.P. (1986). *Glaucoma*. Butterworths, London.
Shields, M.B. (1986). *Textbook of glaucoma*. Williams & Wilkins, Baltimore.

6
Inflammatory eye disease

Uveitis, retinal vasculitis, and scleritis are inflammatory disorders of the ocular tissues which share similar clinical features and an immunologically based aetiology, and are often associated with systemic inflammatory disorders.

Antigen-presenting cells may activate CD4 T lymphocytes inappropriately by presenting autoantigens, leading to an inflammatory response mediated by lymphokines such as interleukin-2, and the macrophage response. Other ocular inflammatory disorders may be based on vasculitic processes caused by deposition of circulating antigen–antibody complexes—in these cases ischaemia (of retina, sclera, or cornea) is an important destructive pathophysiological process.

The initiating trigger in most inflammatory eye disease is not known, though an infective association (virus, *Toxoplasma, Klebsiella*) is implicated in some, while many are associated with specific major histocompatibility complex (MHC) antigens. Uveitis may occur alone, or as a component of retinal vasculitis and scleritis. Concurrent systemic inflammation (systemic lupus erythematosis (SLE), Wegener's granuloma, arthritis, orogenital ulceration) is a common association of inflammatory eye disease.

Uveitis

The uvea is a vascular tissue, derived from mesoderm, which supports the neural components of the eye and the lens. It comprises the iris, ciliary body, and the choroid. Uveitis presents a diversity of clinical types, among which there are several well-defined and consistent patterns and syndromes. The characteristic signs in all types of uveitis are cells and flare in the aqueous and vitreous, and keratic precipitates (KP). Aqueous and vitreous cells are polymorphs and lymphocytes (acute uveitis), and macrophages (chronic uveitis), while KP represent condensations of these cells. Flare is caused by extravasated plasma proteins, indicating increased capillary permeability.

Classification

- anterior uveitis   iritis, iridocyclitis
- intermediate uveitis   pars planitis, chronic cyclitis
- posterior uveitis   chorioretinitis

Uveitis is also classified as granulomatous or non-granulomatous, according to the appearance of the KP (granulomatous KP are fat and globular) and posterior segment signs (choroidal granulomas, or Dalen–Fuchs nodules).

Aetiology

Idiopathic
The pathogenesis of most cases of acute anterior uveitis is not known.

Infections
Uveitis is a feature of some infections, particularly tuberculosis, syphilis, toxo-plasmosis, and leprosy, and it accompanies keratitis and endopthalmitis. A poorly understood connection has been noted between some forms of acute anterior uveitis and acute Gram negative bacterial infections, particularly *Klebsiella*.

MHC antigens
Certain HLA genotypes show strong associations with uveitis and other inflamma-tory disorders (HLA B27 and acute anterior uveitis and ankylosing spondylitis, B5 and Behçet's disease, A29 and birdshot retinochoroidopathy).

Systemic disease
Uveitis is associated with inflammatory disorders of the gut (Crohn's disease and ulcerative colitis), and skin (psoriasis), the joints (ankylosing spondylitis, sero-negative and seropositive arthritis, and juvenile rheumatoid arthritis), the mul-tisystem inflammatory disorders (SLE, PAN, Wegener's granuloma), and Reiter's and Behçet's disease. Uveitis frequently accompanies multiple sclerosis.

Secondary uveitis
Secondary uveitis accompanies keratitis, and other inflammatory, traumatic and ischaemic conditions involving the anterior segment. Chorioretinal inflammation similarly accompanies posterior scleritis.

Masquerade syndromes

Cells and flare may occasionally present with a non-inflammatory primary cause:

- retinal detachment
- intraocular haemorrhage (recent or old)
- ischaemia
- neoplasm   necrotic choroidal melanoma
             retinoblastoma
             metastasis
             lymphoma, leukaemia, reticulum cell sarcoma
- juvenile xanthogranuloma

Anterior uveitis

Symptoms

• pain	dull ache in the eye, and in trigeminal distribution,
• photophobia	caused by pupil spasm,
• reduced vision	due to media clouding or cystoid macular oedema.

Anterior uveitis is sometimes 'silent', causing progressive damage without acute symptoms, but causing serious complications. Posterior synaechia formation, angle damage and risk of pupil block, glaucoma or cataract may be advanced before presentation. Anterior uveitis of this kind is particularly likely in juvenile rheumatoid arthritis (Still's disease), multiple sclerosis, chronic iridocyclitis, and sarcoid. Sustained high pressure, and subsequent glaucomatous damage to the optic nerve, may occur in Fuchs' heterochromic iridocyclitis (HIC).

Signs

1. *Ciliary vessel injection.* Dilated ciliary vessels are densest at the limbus and do not move on gentle manipulation with a cotton wool bud after topical anaesthetic (cf. conjunctivitis).

2. *Miosis.*

3. *KP.* Discrete pearly deposits on the corneal endothelium. Their morphology may suggest aetiology (Table 6.1). KP are densest inferiorly in most anterior uveitis, but in Fuchs' HIC they are distributed more or less evenly over the entire endothelium, including the upper zones. Koeppe and Busacca nodules are large KP on the iris and pupil margin, seen in granulomatous uveitis.

4. *Cells.* Grade white cells in the anterior chamber clinically according to their density (Table 6.2). In anterior uveitis the inflammatory cells are confined to the anterior chamber and anterior vitreous; in cyclitis there are many cells in the anterior vitreous (immediately behind the lens). If there are cells in the posterior vitreous (seen using a fundus lens at the slit-lamp) the patient has posterior uveitis. Vitreous cells are usually concentrated over a focal lesion, or the disc (in papillitis).

5. *Flare.* Plasma protein suspended in aqueous is illuminated as the beam of the

Table 6.1 KP in anterior uveitis

Fine, discrete, smooth	densest inferiorly	idiopathic acute anterior uveitis (AAU)
Variable size, coalescent, extensive	densest inferiorly	severe AAU, often HLA B27 positive, ankylosing spondylitis
Fine or variable, pigmented	densest inferiorly	longstanding. Inactive anterior uveitis (AU).
Medium, round, glistening confluent 'baconfat'	densest inferiorly	Herpes simplex uveitis
Large, globular, greasy-looking 'mutton fat'	densest inferiorly	associated with granulomatous inflammation
Stellate, crenellated	involve upper cornea	Fuchs' HIC

Granulomatous KP are clustered macrophages, while the smaller KP in AAU are predominantly polymorphs.

Table 6.2   Anterior chamber cells in uveitis

Count the cells in a 1.5 × 2 mm slit-lamp beam	
nil	
trace	
+	5–15 cells per field
++	15–50
+++	many

Table 6.3   Anterior chamber flare in uveitis

nil	
trace	
+	faint
++	iris details seen through haze
+++	marked, iris partly obscured
fibrin	intensive protein exudate, sometimes leading to pupillary membrane formation

slit-lamp passes through the anterior chamber (Table 6.3). Plastic uveitis (coagulum of fibrin in anterior chamber) represents more severe exudative reaction than flare (see Table 6.3).

6. *Hypoyon.* In severe uveitis inflammatory cells and fibrin collect as pus in the anterior chamber with an upper fluid level.

7. *Posterior synaechiae (PS).* Adhesions of the posterior iris surface to the lens, indicated by pupil irregularity, especially on dilatation. Pigment deposits on anterior lens surface indicate old PS which have ruptured. Extensive PS formation is typical of HLA B27- and MS-associated acute anterior uveitis.

8. *Intraocular pressure (IOP).* Uveitis usually reduces IOP, reflecting aqueous hyposecretion. IOP may be raised if the trabecular meshwork is significantly obstructed by inflammatory products, or PS cause pupil block.

9. *Lens opacities.* Cataract, typically posterior subcapsular, is common in chronic or recurrent uveitis.

Management

Clinical assessment

Medical history
Identify genitourinary, gastrointestinal, musculoskeletal, respiratory, or dermatological disorder.

Dilated fundus examination
Exclude or identify coexisting posterior segment pathology in anterior uveitis. Vacular sheathing and perivascular 'candlewax dripping' exudates occur in sarcoid, and retinal vascular occlusions indicate Behçet's or SLE. Focal posterior uveitis with pigment epithelial disturbance occurs in toxoplasmosis, birdshot choroido-

retinopathy, and acute multifocal placoid pigment epitheliopathy. Larger, diffuse raised subretinal inflammatory foci occur in tuberculosis and sympathetic ophthalmitis. In intermediate uveitis there is peripheral snowbanking and fluffy vitreous opacities ('cotton wool balls').

Lens opacities are a common complication of uveitis of any aetiology, particularly Fuchs' HIC.

Investigation

Appropriate investigations are suggested by the clinical picture. It is inappropriate to investigate all cases of uveitis with a battery of tests.

Frequent recurrence, severe PS, and an intense anterior chamber reaction are characteristic of HLA B27 uveitis. Request X-rays of the sacro-iliac joints, for evidence of ankylosing spondylitis.

Muttonfat (granulomatous) KP occur in granulomatous disease. Investigate for tuberculosis (TB), syphilis, sarcoid, by: chest X-ray, Mantoux, serology, biochemistry, Kveim (mucosal biopsy may be needed to confirm sarcoid). Exclude *Toxoplasma* or *Toxocara* (particularly in children).

Corneal anaesthesia, baconfat KP (intermediate in size, globular, and translucent), and sector iris atrophy are characteristic of herpes simplex uveitis. Fine scattered amorphous KP occur with corneal anaesthesia in herpes zoster uveitis.

Heterochromia and iris transillumination, together with stellate KP distributed over the entire cornea, are diagnostic of Fuchs' HIC.

Treatment

The aim of treatment is to prevent complications and to give symptomatic relief. Treat with topical steroids to suppress inflammation, and cycloplegia to keep the pupil dilated and reduce iris vessel permeability. This prevents PS formation and relieves photophobia (caused by pupil spasm). Atropine is the most effective cycloplegic, and dexamethasone or prednisolone acetate are the most effective topical steroids; the only advantage in using weaker cycloplegics is the quicker recovery of accommodation when they are discontinued.

Continue treatment for as long as the inflammation is active. Acute anterior uveitis generally lasts for 4–8 weeks, before subsiding completely. Treatment should initially be with frequent topical steroid (as often as hourly for the first week, until the inflammatory signs reduce), reducing subsequently according to the clinical response. Severe cases may require subconjunctival injection of steroid and mydricaine. The patient should be reviewed 2 weeks after all therapy is stopped, and warned to come straight back for immediate treatment at the earliest sign of recurrence.

Complications of anterior uveitis

Complications of the disease

Anterior segment
1. *Posterior synaechia*. Adhesions between the posterior iris and the lens. 360° PS obstruct aqueous circulation through the pupil, leading to iris bombé, angle closure, and secondary glaucoma.

2. *Peripheral anterior synaechiae (PAS)*. Adhesions between the iris root and peripheral cornea. They occlude the drainage angle irreversibly when anterior uveitis is complicated by pupil block and iris bombé.

3. *Cataract*. Recurrent or poorly controlled anterior uveitis is frequently complicated by cataract. Posterior subcapsular lens opacities are typical, and particularly common in Fuchs' HIC.

Posterior segment

Cystoid macular oedema causes reduced acuity. It is less common in anterior than intermediate or posterior uveitis.

Complications caused by steroid treatment

Glaucoma

Steroid-induced glaucoma occurs in 'steroid responders' (5–20 per cent of the population). Treatment with beta-blockers and acetazolamide may be necessary. Raised IOP may limit steroid therapy.

Cataract

Steroid-induced cataractogenesis is dose-related. It follows prolonged use of topical or oral steroid. Patients with chronic uveitis treated with topical steroids for more than a year, and patients inappropriately using topical steroid to relieve external eye symptoms without ophthalmic supervision are particularly at risk.

Herpes virus and fungal infection

Reactivation of herpes simplex keratitis, or stromal invasion by herpes virus, may be facilitated by treatment with topical steroid. It can be difficult to stop steroid treatment of eyes with zoster uveitis without 'rebound' inflammation. Fungal keratitis may, unusually, complicate chronic topical steroid treatment.

Specific uveitis syndromes

HLA B27 positive acute anterior uveitis

Anterior uveitis in HLA B27 individuals is usually intense and recurrent, with severe anterior chamber reaction, often with fibrin exudate (plastic uveitis) and marked PS formation. It is often associated with ankylosing spondylitis or Reiter's syndrome (conjunctivitis, urethritis, polyarthritis, genital ulceration, and low-grade fever). Treat with frequent (initially hourly or 2-hourly) topical steroid and atropine.

Fuchs' heterochromic iridocyclitis

KP are characteristically stellate, with a crinkled outline, and are distributed across the entire corneal endothelium (not confined to the inferior and central zones). PS do not occur. Frank heterochromia is not invariable; more subtle depigmentation of the posterior iris is shown by transillumination. Posterior subcapsular lens opacities and secondary glaucoma are common. Five to 10 per cent of cases are bilateral. Treatment with steroids and cycloplegia is generally not necessary, but IOP must be monitored carefully, and secondary glaucoma treated, using topical beta-blockers, or if these are inadequate by trabeculectomy.

Uveitis secondary to keratitis

Keratitis of any cause is generally associated with secondary anterior uveitis, which should be treated. Cycloplegia (usually atropine) is useful both for symptomatic relief and in preventing complications, but in the presence of active herpes simplex keratitis or acute bacterial ulcer (especially *Pseudomonas*), steroids should be avoided, or used with great care.

Lens-induced uveitis

Lens protein in the anterior chamber causes uveitis, called phacotoxic or phacoanaphylactic. It may be due to incomplete removal of soft lens matter in cataract extraction, or non-surgical trauma. Treat eyes with lens-induced uveitis using topical steroid and mydriatic, and if necessary by surgical removal of the lens remnants.

Herpes simplex and zoster

Uveitis usually complicates herpes simplex keratitis with stromal involvement. Treatment with topical steroids in these eyes may be necessary both to reduce corneal inflammation and also uveitis, but this requires fine judgement and close monitoring; treat also with cycloplegia and acyclovir. Disciform keratitis represents an immunologically mediated endotheliitis associated with herpes simplex, with focal KP and overlying corneal oedema. It responds to treatment with topical steroid.

Herpes zoster uveitis, once treated with local steroids, may flare up when therapy is withdrawn. If the inflammation is mild, cycloplegia alone may suffice. If steroids are necessary, topical treatment may need to be continued, using infrequent dilute steroid (e.g. prednisolone 0.05 per cent twice weekly) for a prolonged period, to prevent recurrent inflammation. Topical acyclovir is claimed by some to be effective in the treatment of zoster, but its action is primarily inhibition of viral replication, rather than anti-inflammatory.

Posner–Schlossman syndrome

Recurrent unilateral uveitis accompanied by raised IOP, which leads to corneal oedema and visual reduction. The inflammatory signs are mild, and the IOP ranges between 30 and 50 mmHg. Treatment with topical steroid to control inflammation lowers IOP, and needs to be continued for several weeks. Posner–Schlossman may be caused by trabeculitis.

Intermediate uveitis (pars planitis)

Intermediate uveitis affects the anterior choroid and ciliary body, with only mild inflammatory signs in the anterior segment. Vitreous cells are associated with deposits in the posterior segment which are mainly peripheral. The eye is usually white and not painful or photophobic. It is commonest in young adults, and usually has a recurrent, protracted natural history, presenting unilaterally with floaters, but both eyes are affected in up to 75 per cent.

Signs

'Snowballs' or 'cotton wool balls'—small fluffy vitreous inflammatory foci, at the extreme periphery, sometimes accompanied by accumulation of inflammatory cells and exudate, as 'snowbanks'. The signs are most marked inferiorly, and can be accompanied by dense cellular vitritis and fibrous organization. Cystoid macular oedema may occur secondary to the inflammation. Fluorescein angiography shows diffuse leakage from retinal veins and capillaries.

Indications for treatment

- cystoid macular oedema,
- intense vitritis and fibrous organization,
- cataract.

Treatment

Most cases can be monitored untreated, unless cystoid macular oedema develops. Treat if necessary using oral steroids, or with orbital floor or sub-Tenon injection of soluble or depo-steroid. Cataract extraction may be necessary if there is significant lens opacification.

Posterior uveitis

Toxoplasma retinitis

Ocular infection by *Toxoplasma gondii* causes retinitis, with secondary involvement of the choroid, and is a relatively common cause of chorioretinal scarring. Typically there are satellite lesions, which may be active, around old scars with central atrophy and marginal pigment clumping. Active lesions have indistinct creamy raised edges with overlying vitreous inflammatory cells. Serology is specific, but is generally unhelpful, and the diagnosis is made on the basis of clinical findings.

Natural history

Toxoplasmosis may be a congenital or an acquired infection, usually arising from ingestion of material infected by the oocyst of *T. gondii* derived from animal flesh or faeces. Its systemic phase gives rise to a limited febrile illness, during which any tissue may become infected. Congenital (transplacental) infection has a range of results. It may cause spontaneous abortion, brain damage with convulsions and cerebral calcification, retinochoroiditis, hepatosplenomegaly, or may be subclinical. Acquired toxoplasmosis has a similarly variable effect, but CNS involvement is typical of infection in immunosuppressed patients, including those with AIDS.

Clinical features of ocular toxoplasmosis
Ocular toxoplasmosis presents with floaters and reduced vision, due to inflammatory cells in the vitreous. There are mild to moderate anterior segment signs of inflammation, with KP that may appear granulomatous or non-granulomatous. The punched out chorioretinal lesions seen on indirect ophthalmoscopy are characteristic, and usually diagnostic. Recurrences occur at the edge of scars, as the inactive bradyzoite form reverts to become active tachyzoites. Serious visual damage occurs if the macular, papillomacular bundle, or disc become involved.

Treatment
1. Watch and wait if there is no threat to the macula, papillomacular bundle, or disc.
2. Treat with cycloplegia and topical steroid if there is marked activity in the anterior chamber.
3. Treat with oral steroids, with or without antimicrobial therapy (clindamycin 300 mg, q.d.s. for 2–4 weeks, or pyrimethamine 25 mg daily, sulphadiazine and plate for 4 weeks, monitoring fbc weekly), if the macula or disc are threatened. Pyrimethamine may cause aplastic anaemia, and clindamycin may cause pseudomembranous colitis.

Antimicrobial therapy has not been shown to be useful if macula and disc are not threatened.

Sarcoid

Sarcoid is associated with a focal or diffuse choroiditis, with vasculitis, sheathing, and perivascular 'candlewax dripping' exudates, and anterior chamber signs of granulomatous uveitis. Diagnosis is made by chest X-ray (CXR), raised serum calcium, Kveim and mucosal biopsy. Treat with oral steroids, in conjunction with a physician.

TB and syphilis

Syphilis causes signs of granulomatous uveitis, but may take any inflammatory form in the posterior segment. Miliary TB presents with multifocal subretinal inflammatory foci, and syphilis often leaves widespread retinal pigment epithelium changes, with pigment clumping or scattering. Unusual presentations of granulomatous uveitis should be tested for TB and syphilis by CXR, serology, and further investigation as necessary.

Behçet's disease

This produces bilateral signs in both anterior and posterior segments. There is an obliterative retinal vasculitis, with branch vein occlusion, causing retinal haemorrhages and cotton wool spots.
   It is associated with:

- oral ulceration,
- erythema nodosum,

- genital ulceration,
- polyarthritis.

Vasculitis and vein occlusion in the posterior segment threaten vision if uncontrolled. Treatment requires oral steroids, sometimes with immunosuppressants (azathioprine and cyclosporin). Areas of retina made ischaemic by vein occlusion may be treated with scatter photocoagulation, to prevent neovascularization.

AIDS and cytomegalovirus (CMV) retinitis

CMV posterior uveitis is only seen in severely immunocompromised patients, and is most commonly seen in established AIDS. There is rapid and profound visual loss, caused by a widespread haemorrhagic ischaemic retinitis, with extensive cotton wool spots, and deep and superficial retinal haemorrhages. The appearance of ischaemic signs and retinal haemorrhages is sometimes likened to that of a pizza. There may also be optic neuritis, or concurrent CNS involvement.

Vogt–Koyanagi–Harada syndrome

A rare combination of posterior uveitis, serous retinal detachment and encephalitis, with vitiligo, alopecia, and poliosis (white lashes).

Sympathetic ophthalmitis

Sympathetic ophthalmitis is a rare bilateral chronic granulomatous uveitis which follows perforating ocular trauma with uveal disruption. Its onset is variable, usually from 4–8 weeks to 1 year after injury, and its destructive course may last weeks, months, or years. The signs are a granulomatous anterior uveitis with vitreous cells, and characteristic discrete pale patches at the level of the retinal pigment epithelium called Dalen–Fuchs nodules. Treatment requires topical and systemic steroids; recently these have been supplemented in some cases by specific inhibition of T lymphocytes, using cyclosporin, with reported good effect.

Retinal vasculitis

Retinal vasculitis occurs either as an isolated ocular disorder, or as a component of a systemic autoimmune vasculitis (Table 6.4). The underlying pathology is caused by immune complex deposition on the basement membrane of retinal veins. These immune complexes are based on antibodies to either ocular (e.g. retinal S antigen) or non-ocular antigens. Cell-mediated immunity, based on T lymphocytes and activated macrophages, is also important in some (Wegener's granulomatosis, sarcoid). An infectious agent is associated with the inflammation in some, notably CMV in AIDS.

Signs

Foci of inflammation around retinal vessels appear as cuffing, sheathing, or occlusion. The surrounding retina is often involved in the inflammatory process,

Table 6.4   Retinal vasculitis: aetiology

Retinal vasculitis without a non-ocular component
  Eales' disease
  Acute retinal necrosis
  Sympathetic ophthalmitis
Systemic inflammatory disorders featuring retinal vasculitis
  SLE
  Polyarteritis nodosa
  Wegener's granulomatosis
  Sarcoid
  Behçet's disease
  Multiple sclerosis
  CMV retinitis (especially in AIDS)
  TB
  Syphilis

and the retina distal to the site of an occlusive vasculopathy is ischaemic, with haemorrhages and cotton wool spots. Inflamed retinal vessels leak on fluorescein angiography, as do vessels passing through areas of ischaemic retina. Secondary effects of the inflammatory reaction and consequent ischaemia include cystoid macular oedema, retinal neovascularization, epiretinal membrane formation, and tractional or exudative retinal detachment.

Signs of posterior uveitis occur in eyes with retinal vasculitis, and it is difficult to identify the primary pathophysiological process in diseases exhibiting signs of both processes, such as sympathetic ophthalmitis, sarcoid, and Behçet's disease.

Investigation and treatment

Retinal vasculitis is a potentially blinding condition, management of which requires collaboration between the ophthalmologists and a physician specializing in inflammatory disorders. Possible systemic associations must be investigated, and therapy is based on systemic modulation of the immune response.

Initial treatment with high dose ('pulse') intravenous steroid therapy is advocated by some authorities, with subsequent sustained immunosuppression using oral steroids, and cyclosporin to reduce T-cell activity.

Specific antimicrobial or antiviral therapy may be indicated if there is an underlying infection (TB or CMV). The management of CMV retinopathy in patients with AIDS requires experience and interdisciplinary collaboration. Antiviral agents are not curative and require intravenous administration over a prolonged period, while CNS involvement may already be established when the patient presents with retinal involvement.

Scleritis (see p. 48)

Scleritis is a non-infective inflammatory disorder of sclera which is generally associated with other manifestations of immunologically mediated inflammatory disease, particularly rheumatoid, SLE, PAN, and Wegener's granulomatosis; it is occasionally related to previous eye surgery. Its course is characteristically chronic and destructive, and its management requires immunomodulation using systemic therapy.

Presentation

Scleritis presents with severe pain in and around the eye, which often radiates through the forehead; there may be associated photophobia and watering. Vision is impaired if the posterior sclera is involved (due to macular oedema or exudative detachment), or if limbal involvement causes simultaneous corneal disease (ulceration or melting). Involved sclera is thickened and diffusely red or purplish in colour, but the pattern of individual normal vessels is often not distinguishable. These signs are best seen in natural daylight, and may not be visible using the slit-lamp or in inadequate artificial light. As the disease progresses the sclera may become thinned, or perforate (necrotizing scleritis), revealing underlying choroid.

Assessment and investigation

Slit-lamp examination is an important part of the assessment of scleritis, since cells in the anterior chamber or vitreous indicate the presence of an inflammatory disorder which is not confined to the surface of the eye, and IOP may be raised, either by the scleritis or its treatment. Examine also with red-free light to demonstrate avascular regions of sclera. Ultrasound examination (B-scan with measurement by vector A-scan) shows the thickness of the posterior sclera, which is an important objective sign in monitoring progress and response to treatment.

Check full blood count, especially for white cells and differential, and erythrocyte sedimentation rate; anti-neutrophil cytoplasm antibody (ANCA); autoantibody screen (antinuclear factor, rheumatoid factor, C-reactive protein); CXR, and manage coexisting systemic disease in conjunction with a physician or rheumatologist.

Treatment

Mild cases of scleritis may respond to non-steroidal anti-inflammatory agents (indomethacin, flurbiprofen).

The treatment of more serious scleritis requires experience both of the condition itself, and of the immunosuppressive agents which are often required. Some authorities begin treatment with high-dose 'pulsed' intravenous methylprednisolone, followed by maintenance on oral steroids in high dose; cyclosporin A may be used to supplement steroid in suppressing the immune response. If perforation threatens, scleral or corneoscleral graft may save the eye, but these cases generally have a poor prognosis. Topical treatment alone is inadequate in the management of active scleritis, but topical steroid and atropine are necessary to suppress concurrent anterior uveitis.

Recommended further reading

Kanski, J.J. (1987). *Uveitis. A colour manual of diagnosis and treatment*. Butterworths, London.
Michelson, J.B. (1989). *A colour atlas of uveitis diagnosis*. Wolfe, London.
Nussenblatt, R.B. & Palestine, A. (1989). *Uveitis. Fundamentals and clinical practice*. Year Book Medical Publishing, Chicago.

7

The orbit

Anatomy

The orbit is a pyramidal cavity, with its open base anteriorly and its apex posteriorly. The medial walls of the right and left orbit are parallel, and their lateral walls make an angle of 90° with each other, and 45° with the sagittal midline. The bony walls of the orbit are lined with periosteum called the periorbita, which is continuous anteriorly, at the rim of the orbit, with the orbital septum. This is inserted into the tarsal plates, bounding the orbit anteriorly.

Table 7.1 Orbit: walls and relations

	Components	Relations	Structures
Floor (roof of maxillary antrum)	maxillary palatine zygomatic	maxillary antrum	infraorbital nerve
Roof (floor of frontal sinus)	frontal sphenoid lr wing	anterior cranial fossa frontal sinus	lacrimal gland fossa superior oblique trochlea
Medial wall	ethmoid maxillary lacrimal sphenoid	ethmoid air cells sphenoid sinus	lacrimal sac fossa
Lateral wall	zygomatic sphenoid gr wing	temporal fossa middle cranial fossa	Whitnall's ligament pterygopalatine fossa

Table 7.2 Orbit: openings

	Structures	Communication
Optic foramen	optic nerve ophthalmic artery sympathetics	middle cranial fossa
Superior orbital fissure (SOF)	III, IV, V_1 and VI ophthalmic veins	cavernous sinus
Inferior orbital fissure	V_2 communicating veins	pterygoid plexus
Lacrimal sac fossa	nasolacrimal duct	inferior meatus

The orbital septum separates inflammation into preseptal (involving the lids only) and postseptal (involving the orbital cavity) compartments. Postseptal pathology may involve the eye, the optic nerve, and by extension through the SOF and the optic foramen, the cavernous sinus and brain.

The rectus muscles are invested by a fibrous sheet, which joins their margins as the intermuscular septum to form an enclosed space. Structures and pathology within this sheath are called intraconal, and those outside are extraconal. The sheath is continuous with Tenon's capsule, and at the orbital apex it is condensed as the tendinous ring of Zinn, to which are also joined the periorbita and the optic nerve sheath.

The distinction between pre- and postseptal, and intra- and extraconal pathology is clinically important in the assessment of orbital disease.

Pathology

The intraorbital tissues include the rectus and oblique muscles and their sheaths, orbital fat and blood vessels, lymphoid tissue, lacrimal gland and the upper part of the lacrimal drainage system, III, IV, V_1, VI, sympathetics and para-sympathetics and the ciliary ganglion, as well as the eye and optic nerve. Orbital disease is caused by malformation, inflammation or neoplasia in these tissues. It occurs as primary disease, or follows local invasion (from the lids, paranasal sinuses, nasopharynx, brain, or dura), or haematogenous spread from a distant primary infective or neoplastic focus. The orbital septum acts as a barrier to infection spreading backwards into the orbit from a lid infection.

Clinical presentation of orbital disease

Symptoms

The nature of symptoms suggest how orbital tissues may be involved in disease:

- diplopia ⠀⠀ocular displacement, muscle restriction
- pain ⠀⠀⠀⠀deep, boring: tumour, inflammation
  ⠀⠀⠀⠀⠀⠀gritty discomfort: thyroid eye disease
  ⠀⠀⠀⠀⠀⠀worse on eye movement: extraocular muscles involved
- visual loss ⠀optic nerve involvement
- lid swelling ⠀inflammation or tumour
- sensory loss ⠀V_1 and V_2 involvement

If structures outside the orbit are involved, symptoms may include:

- epistaxis, obstruction, anosmia (nasopharyngeal involvement),
- headache, congestion, discharge (paranasal sinus involvement),
- epilepsy, endocrine disturbance (brain and pituitary involvement).

Signs

Orbital disease produces extraocular, intraocular, and functional signs.

Extraocular signs

Focal swelling or mass

Lacrimal gland mass presents in the upper outer quadrant. It can often be palpated on the orbital rim, and its posterior edge cannot be defined. Dermoid may present in any location, most commonly the upper outer orbit. It is smooth, soft, and fluctuant.

Proptosis

Dysthyroid ophthalmopathy is the commonest cause of proptosis in adults.

Measurement of proptosis

Record the prominence of each eye from the lateral orbital margin in mm, using the Hertel exophthalmometer; the separation between the arms of the instrument must be noted, for future comparison. The normal range is taken as 18–24 mm, but asymmetry >2 mm, and increasing proptosis over time, are more significant signs.

Characteristics of proptosis

Proptosis indicates that at least part of the mass must lie behind the equator, and may be axial or asymmetric. Axial proptosis suggests an intraconal mass, usually dysthyroid, cavernous haemangioma or optic nerve tumour. Asymmetric proptosis causes horizontal or vertical displacement, and is due to an extraconal mass, causing displacement superiorly (maxillary sinus tumour), inferonasally (lacrimal gland tumour) or inferolaterally (frontal or ethmoid mucocoele or abscess).

Bilateral proptosis occurs in dysthyroid ophthalmopathy, lymphoma, pseudo-tumour, metastatic disease, leukaemia, caroticocavernous fistula, and cavernous sinus thrombosis.

Pulsation indicates a mass in communication with the internal carotid artery or a posterior bony defect, and a bruit indicates an arteriovenous communication (usually caroticocavernous fistula).

Pseudoproptosis

A misleading appearance of proptosis may be caused by:

- high myopia,
- buphthalmos,
- dysthyroid lagophthalmos,
- shallow orbit (craniofacial dysostosis),
- facial asymmetry,
- contralateral enophthalmos.

Retinoscopy confirms myopia; old photographs and inspection of the whole face will help confirm developmental malformation.

Retropulsion

The resistance to pressing the eye back into the orbit reveals the consistency of a retrobulbar mass. A fluid-filled structure (cyst or vascular malformation) is yielding; solid tumours resist retropulsion.

Ocular motility

Restriction of movement, squint, and diplopia may have a mechanical (inflammation, entrapment, fibrosis) or a neurogenic cause. Test eye movements to the six cardinal positions, and chart them objectively on the Lees screen, so that the developing picture can be accurately monitored.

Mechanical restriction of movement may be combined with ocular displacement, and can be confirmed by a traction test (move the eye in the restricted field with forceps holding the Tenon's capsule adjacent to the limbus, after topical anaesthesia); resistance occurs in an eye whose muscles are restricted). Diffuse restriction implies a more general mass effect, or splinting of the optic nerve (e.g. by optic nerve sheath meningioma).

Bilateral global restriction of eye movements is caused by ocular myopathy (external ophthalmoplegia), or pseudo-ophthalmoplegia (supranuclear gaze paresis). The two are distinguished by reflex movements (Bell's phenomenon, doll's head manoeuvre, and response to caloric stimulation). Reflex responses are preserved in supranuclear gaze paresis, but absent in ocular myopathy.

Testing eye movements can help to distinguish pre- and postseptal inflammation, when lid swelling prevents direct examination of the affected eye. The pursuit movements of an eye whose extraocular muscles are inflamed are restricted, as are the conjugate movements of the more easily observed unaffected eye.

Conjunctiva and lids

External signs of orbital inflammation occur unless disease is confined entirely to the orbital apex. Rhabdomyosarcoma presents with marked external inflammatory signs, together with proptosis and cervical lymphadenopathy.

Thyroid eye disease causes chemosis and conjunctival injection over the rectus muscles, as well as lid lag and incomplete lid closure (lagophthalmos). S-shaped deformity of the upper lid suggests orbital involvement in neurofibromatosis. There is often patchy bruising beneath the lower lid in neuroblastoma.

Intraocular signs

Optic disc

Disc swelling indicates optic nerve compression or orbital apex congestion. In dysthyroid ophthalmopathy, disc swelling suggests raised intraorbital pressure, for which decompressive measures must be considered.

Disc pallor and optic atrophy are caused by established compressive optic neuropathy or posterior ciliary vessel occlusion.

Retinal vessels

Tortuosity, or occlusion with retinal haemorrhages, is caused by compression of the central retinal vein. Slowly progressive occlusion of the central retinal vein, caused by optic nerve compression (classically by optic nerve sheath meningioma) leads to the development of an opticociliary shunt (an abnormal dilated venous channel draining the retinal circulation through the edge of the disc).

Choroidal folds

Radial or concentric corrugations of the choroid and overlying retina at the posterior pole are signs of a retrobulbar mass. Fundus fluorescein angiography shows alternating bands of hyper- and hypofluorescence.

Intraocular pressure (IOP)

Increased IOP on elevation indicates inferior rectus restriction. This occurs typically in orbit blowout fracture and dysthyroid ophthalmopathy.

Functional signs

Pupil

Relative afferent pupil defect (RAPD) indicates compromised optic nerve function. Orbital causes of optic neuropathy include tumour compressing or arising in the optic nerve or its sheath, or compressive optic neuropathy due to raised intraorbital pressure, for example in dysthyroid ophthalmopathy.

Visual field

Focal invasion of the optic nerve is shown by field testing. The fields of both eyes should always be plotted, to reveal signs of bilateral involvement.

Investigation of orbital disease

Radiology

The most appropriate radiological technique by which to investigate a particular clinical problem is best identified by discussion between clinician and radiologist.

Plain films

Plain skull radiographs can be used to demonstrate the orbital walls, lacrimal gland fossa, sphenoid ridge, and paranasal sinuses. They also show abnormal calcification, such as occurs in retinoblastoma, meningioma, varices and choroidal osteoma, as well as the hyperostosis seen in sphenoid ridge meningioma. The four standard views which are particularly helpful in demonstrating orbital pathology are:

Lateral
- Structures: pituitary fossa and nasopharynx.

Caldwell
- structures   superior and lateral orbital rim
                 medial orbital wall
                 ethmoid and frontal sinuses
- geometry   plate perpendicular to canthomeatal line
                 tube angled down at 25° to canthomeatal line

Waters
- structures   orbit roof and floor (for blowout fracture)
- geometry   plate perpendicular to tube
                 tube angled 37° above canthomeatal line

Submento-vertex
- structures   sphenoid and ethmoid sinuses, nasopharynx
- geometry   hyperextended neck, plate parallel to canthomeatal line
                 tube perpendicular to plate

CT

Computerized imaging gives high quality three-dimensional views of the orbits and their contents, and is routinely undertaken to define both bony and soft tissue abnormalities in the orbit. It is particularly useful in the investigation of trauma, proptosis, orbital mass and inflammation, and sinus disease, and has superseded plain radiography in the imaging of the optic canal.

Standard CT scans give a transverse section, but other views can be obtained by positioning the patient, or by computerized reformatting. Enhancement of the image by the use of intravenous radio-opaque dye, increases contrast between vascular and non-vascular structures.

MRI

MRI gives high definition images of soft tissue structures, but is less useful than CT in imaging bone involvement.

Angiography

Venography may be useful in defining orbital varices and the cavernous sinus. Arteriography shows aneurysm and arteriovenous communication. The indications for angiography have become fewer since CT scanning, which is non-invasive, has become widely available.

Biopsy

Biopsy, followed by immunohistochemical staining, may be necessary to diagnose definitively the various forms of lymphoma, and to distinguish these from reactive lymphoid hyperplasia.

Orbital disorders

The range of orbital diseases which affect children differs from those affecting adults. The more common of these are listed in Table 7.3.

Table 7.3   Orbital disorders

Orbital disorders in children	
Congenital	microphthalmos, anophthalmos, orbital cyst
	craniofacial development malformation
Infection	preseptal cellulitis
	orbital cellulitis
Tumour	dermoid cyst
	capillary haemangioma (strawberry naevus)
	neural tumours
	optic nerve glioma
	neurofibroma
	rhabdomyosarcoma
	neuroblastoma
	leukaemia

Orbital disorders in adults	
Endocrine	dysthyroid eye disease
Inflammation	infective
	preseptal and orbital cellulitis
	non-infective
	pseudotumour
	Wegener's granuloma
Tumour	cavernous haemangioma, orbital varices
	neural tumours
	nerve sheath meningioma
	optic nerve glioma
	lacrimal tumours
	benign pleomorphic
	malignant pleomorphic
	adenocarcinoma
	lymphoid tumours
	benign ('reactive')
	malignant (lymphoma)
	secondary tumours
	lid
	eye
	sinus
	intracranial
	metastatic (breast, lung, prostate)

Dysthyroid eye disease

Dysthryroid eye disease is the commonest cause of unilateral proptosis in adults (due to asymmetric, not unilateral disease). It is most common in females (F:M = 8:1), and in middle age. All orbital tissues, particularly the extraocular muscles, are involved in the chronic inflammatory process. Management requires medical correction of endocrine status, and monitoring the eye disease:

- muscle imbalance and angle of deviation,
- proptosis (exophthalmometer),
- cornea for exposure keratopathy,
- RAPD and fields for optic nerve compression.

Clinical features and management

Motility

Restriction of eye movements, and consequent diplopia, is initially caused by stimulation of extraocular muscles (phase of contraction); they later undergo fibrosis (phase of contracture). Inferior rectus is most commonly involved, causing restriction of elevation. The deviation may be unstable for months during the active phase of the inflammation, during which time it is corrected using temporary Fresnel prisms applied to spectacle lenses. Once stable, surgical correction may be planned.

Botulinum toxin-induced paresis of the anatagonist is sometimes used to reduce a large deviation, and to reduce the secondary contracture of the antagonist.

Proptosis

This is measured using the exophthalmometer, and provides an objective measure of the clinical course of the disease. Sight-threatening orbital congestion may be present without progressive proptosis, if the tissues of the orbital septum are unyielding.

Exposure

Caused by proptosis and lagophthalmos. Monitor the cornea carefully for signs of exposure (Rose Bengal staining), and treat with lubricants, ointment, or tarsorrhaphy. Treat lagophthalmos which is sufficient to cause or threaten significant keratopathy by tarsorrhaphy, or extension of levator aponeurosis using scleral graft or mersilene mesh implant.

Orbital congestion

Raised intraorbital pressure is caused by inflammation within the confined space of the orbit. The optic nerve circulation may be compromised, and optic nerve function must be monitored (visual acuity and field, relative afferent pupil reaction, optic disc appearance). Orbit decompression may be achieved surgically, or by treatment with steroids, immunomodulation, or radiotherapy.

Differential diagnosis

- orbital tumour,
- myasthenia,
- motor nerve palsies.

Investigation

The relationship between clinical and biochemical thyroid disorder is variable. T_3 and T_4 may be raised, normal or decreased. The most consistent biochemical abnormalities are immunological; anti-thyroglobulin and thyroid microsome antibodies are usually present.

CT scan of orbits confirms fusiform swelling of extraocular muscles.

Orbital inflammation

Acute orbital inflammation

Cellulitis involving lid and orbital tissues is divided anatomically into preseptal and postseptal compartments by the orbital septum, which joins the orbital rim with the tarsal plate. Orbital and preseptal inflammation can be distinguished clinically by observing eye movements to pursuit, which are full if the inflammation is preseptal, but restricted in both eyes in postseptal cellulitis.

Orbital cellulitis must be treated vigorously and monitored carefully, because of the danger of spread of infection through the orbital veins into the cavernous sinus, leading to cavernous sinus thrombosis.

Preseptal cellulitis

Swelling of lid tissues which is rapid and severe, on account of the loose subcutaneous tissues, and may make examination of the eye difficult. Preseptal cellulitis usually begins as a superficial infection which rapidly extends to involve upper and lower lids. It may spread into the orbit via the angular vein, which is an anastamotic communication between the facial and orbital veins. Culture conjunctival and nasopharyngeal swabs, and blood if the response to treatment is poor. The infecting organism is usually *Staphylococcus*, or sometimes *Haemophilus* in children. Treat with broad spectrum antibiotic—a cephalosporin, or ampicillin/flucloxacillin.

Orbital (postseptal) cellulitis

Presentation is with painful proptosis, chemosis, fever, headache, and ophthalmoplegia. Visual impairment and RAPD indicate optic nerve involvement at the orbital apex, which mandates urgent vigorous treatment. Orbital cellulitis usually originates from the ethmoid, sphenoid, or frontal sinus, or the lacrimal sac, either by direct extension, bony destruction, or through veins. Extension through the ophthalmic veins into the cavernous sinus can be rapid, causing cavernous sinus thrombosis, meningitis, and cerebral abscess.

Sinus X-rays show opacification in the infected sinus, and CT may show overlying periosteal elevation, indicating a subperiosteal abscess. An ENT opinion should be arranged to confirm sinus disease, and if necessary to drain the infected sinus surgically. Conjunctival swabs and pus should be Gram stained and cultured. The infection is usually bacterial, and requires in-patient treatment with intravenous antibiotics and surgical drainage if there is a localized abscess. Occasionally herpes virus (simplex or zoster) may cause orbital cellulitis.

Cavernous sinus thrombosis

This serious complication of orbital inflammation causes visual reduction, pupil dilatation, disc swelling with retinal vein obstruction, and ophthalmoplegia. It requires immediate vigorous treatment with intravenous antibiotics in high dose, including penicillinase-resistant and anti-Gram negative agents.

Pseudotumour (orbital inflammatory syndrome)

Pseudotumour, Tolosa–Hunt, and the orbital inflammatory syndrome all describe chronic lymphocytic inflammation in the orbit, which is of uncertain cause, and may be impossible to distinguish clinically from lymphoma. The condition may affect the orbital tissues diffusely, or more focally involve the superior orbital fissure (Tolosa–Hunt syndrome), the anterior cavernous sinus or the optic canal; it may be complicated by posterior scleritis and exudative retinal detachment. It is usually unilateral, bilateral orbital involvement suggesting a proliferative disorder or systemic vasculitis.

Presentation

- pain: acute severe, boring;
- vessels: diffuse ciliary and conjunctival engorgement.

Neurological signs — according to the location:

- SOF   III, IV, V_1, and VI signs
               painful diplopia, ptosis,
               decreased corneal sensation
- optic foramen   visual impairment
               RAPD
               Horner's syndrome

Investigation

1. Exclude a focal tumour; CT and ultrasound confirm the diffuse distribution of the inflammation, and narrowing of the SOF or optic canal in the orbital apex syndromes.
2. Biopsy anterior lesions for immunohistochemical study.
3. Arrange medical examination and appropriate radiological examination to exclude remote lymphoma.

Differential diagnosis

Painful ophthalmoplegia may also be caused by diabetes, aneurysm, meningitis, cavernous sinus thrombosis, systemic vasculitis, and intracranial tumour.

Orbital inflammation may be due specifically to vasculitis (giant cell arteritis PAN, Wegener's granuloma), or sarcoid (with lacrimal gland involvement and uveitis).

Treatment

Treatment with systemic steroids, supplemented by cyclosporin A if necessary, produces rapid resolution.

Cysts

Dermoid, mucocoele, and encephalocoele

Dermoid is a developmental cyst caused by inclusion of ectoderm into the mesodermal tissues of the orbit. It is usually located in the superotemporal orbit or brow, and usually presents at the surface without causing proptosis. Orbital dermoid is generally of cosmetic significance, but it may rupture, causing acute orbital inflammation.

Mucocoeles derive from adjacent sinuses (frontal, ethmoid, or sphenoid) by erosion of bone. They cause proptosis, and neurological signs according to involvement of the optic and ocular motor nerves.

Encephalocoeles are uncommon developmental forebrain anomalies. It is important to avoid attempting to excise an orbital encephalocoele (which can be identified by radiological demonstration of a bony defect) in the mistaken belief that it is a dermoid, since encephalocoele communicates with the brain.

Vascular lesions

Haemangioma

Orbital haemangiomas in childhood are usually of the capillary type. They present as a 'strawberry naevus', often extending into the lids and on to the face, which grows during the first year of life, but usually regresses spontaneously by the age of 5 or 6 years.

They are ill-defined, and are not amenable to surgical excision. Because of their tendency to spontaneous regression they are best treated with reassurance and non-intervention unless, rarely, they cause amblyopia by obstructing the visual axis, when some involution can be encouraged with intralesional injection of depomedrone. More commonly amblyopia is associated with anisometropia or astigmatism; for this reason the acuities and refractions in children with orbital haemangiomas should be monitored.

Haemangioma presenting in adults is cavernous, presenting as slowly increasing painless proptosis or ocular displacement which can be reduced by firm pressure; choroidal folds; and signs of optic nerve compression. Orbit X-ray shows calcified phleboliths, demonstrated on ultrasound as echogenic foci in a non-echogenic background. Cavernous haemangioma is encapsulated, and can be excised surgically.

Carotico-cavernous fistula (CCF) and dural shunt

CCF is an artery–vein shunt, which usually follows trauma, but may occur spontaneously in atherosclerotic or congenitally malformed internal carotid arteries. The communication raises the pressure in the cavernous sinus, and therefore also in the orbital veins. The episcleral, conjunctival, and retinal vessels are dilated, there may be pulsatile proptosis, and a bruit is present on auscultating the eye. Complications include retinal haemorrhage, disc oedema, and glaucoma. CCF is closed off by balloon embolization under radiological control.

Dural shunts are spontaneous abnormal communications, at lower pressure than CCF, from the smaller dural vessels, in arteriopaths.

Orbital varices

Abnormally dilated orbital veins cause transient non-pulsatile proptosis, which is easily reduced by sustained firm pressure. Proptosis is most marked on lying down or Valsalva, when the varices become filled with blood. Plain radiographs show calcification within the varices.

Tumours

Optic nerve tumours

Signs

Proptosis, eye movement restriction, reduced acuity, RAPD, pale disc, optico-ciliary shunt vessels, and loss of definition of the orbital margin.

Optic nerve sheath meningioma

Meningiomas are commoner in females than males, and reach a peak incidence in the seventh decade. Optic nerve sheath meningioma is often an extension of a cranial dural meningioma, but may arise *de novo*. Though adults are affected most commonly, the tumour is more rapidly growing in children, in whom it is sometimes associated with neurofibromatosis. Anterior tumours cause proptosis, while those involving the orbital apex and optic canal affect vision early. There is typically radiological hyperostosis of adjacent bone. Surgery seldom saves sight, because optic nerve vessels are inevitably damaged, but may be indicated to try to arrest spread to the fellow optic nerve.

Optic nerve glioma

Optic nerve glioma affects children most commonly, and is frequently (but not exclusively) associated with neurofibromatosis and tuberous sclerosis. Visual function (acuity, colour vision and field) is reduced early. Intracanalicular glioma causes radiological enlargement of the optic canal, and the tumours are demonstrated well by CT scan.

Treatment is by radiotherapy or local resection of involved optic nerve (to reduce proptosis).

Lacrimal gland tumours

Lacrimal tumours present with eccentric proptosis, the eye displaced downwards and nasally, and a mass palpable in the lacrimal fossa. The fossa is radiologically enlarged, benign tumours causing smooth enlargement, and malignant tumours eroding bone.

Malignancy and invasiveness are variable, according to cellular pattern. Benign swelling may be essentially lymphocytic inflammation, or may resemble pleomorphic salivary tumours, which sometimes become malignant. Malignant lacrimal tumours are generally adenocarcinomas.

Treatment is by biopsy, followed if necessary by surgical excision, orbital exenteration, and radiotherapy.

Rhabdomyosarcoma

The commonest orbital primary in children, with average age of presentation of 7 years. There is rapidly growing eccentric (usually inferotemporal) unilateral proptosis, loss of definition of the orbital margin, soft tissue swelling, and injected blood vessels, suggesting acute inflammation. A suspected rhabdomyosarcoma should be imaged by CT and biopsied without delay; management includes examination of lymph nodes, chest X-ray, bone marrow examination, and lumbar puncture, to exclude metastasis. Treatment is by combined radiotherapy and chemotherapy.

Neuroblastoma

An uncommon metastatic tumour derived from the sympathetic chain, which presents as rapidly increasing ocular displacement and proptosis, associated with periorbital bruising, in infants. Diagnosis is by CT of the orbits as well as the abdomen and mediastinum, to demonstrate the primary tumour.

Leukaemia

The orbits are sometimes involved in advanced leukaemia, particularly acute lymphatic leukaemia.

Secondary tumours

Adults

Metastatic tumours derive from lung, breast, prostate, bowel and kidney. Tumours of the paranasal sinuses and the nasopharynx invade the orbit directly. X-ray indicates sinus or nasopharyngeal pathology, and these tumours are confirmed by biopsy, in conjunction with ENT consultation. Treatment of orbital secondary tumours is by radiotherapy.

Children

Neuroblastoma, osteosarcoma, and leukaemia are the commonest secondary tumours in children. Osteosarcoma presents later than neuroblastoma, and leukaemia at any age.

Recommended further reading

Char, D. (1990). *Thyroid eye disease*, 2nd edn. Churchill Livingstone, New York.
Rootman, J. (1988). *Diseases of the orbit*. J.B. Lippincott, Philadelphia.

8
Neuro-ophthalmology

The visual system provides mankind's largest and most highly organized sensory input, with more afferent fibres than all the other sensory systems combined. Eye movements must be accurately co-ordinated, and extremely precise, to fixate, follow and refixate an object of regard, in order to make most efficient use of the sensory potential of the visual system. Neuro-ophthalmology describes the pathways and central mechanisms which subserve these sensory and motor functions, and the disorders which affect them.

The sensory pathway projects from the outer segments of the receptors, via the retinal ganglion cells, to the optic nerves and the chiasm. Here the nasal fibres from each eye decussate, and the pathway becomes arranged into hemifields. The optic tracts leave the chiasm, containing fibres from both eyes, and project to the lateral geniculate nuclei (LGN) where they relay. Binocular interaction first occurs at the LGN, which is made up of six lamellae (three from each eye). LGN cells remain monocular (one cell receives input from only one eye), but cells with the same visual projection are located in corresponding positions in adjacent lamellae. Fibres from the LGN project to the occipital cortex as the optic radiations, and also to other cortical areas via association fibres. Incompletely understood, and phylogenetically more ancient, secondary pathways project to subcortical nuclei and the thalamus.

The motor system is based in the brainstem. The ocular motor nuclei innervate the internal and external eye muscles through the motor nerves III, IV, and VI, receiving their input from the gaze centres and the cerebellum. The brainstem gaze centres, in turn, integrate descending inputs from the visual and frontal cortex (controlling visually directed and voluntary movements) with vestibular input (co-ordinating eye and head movement) and eye position information (feedback from the extraocular muscle proprioceptors). They generate fast and slow eye movements, by determining the patterns of innervation fed into the motor nuclei, to produce agonist contraction and antagonist inhibition in the two eyes, and an appropriate binocular movement.

Visual function depends on accurate eye positioning by the motor system, and accurate eye-positioning requires visually mediated control.

Neuro-ophthalmic assessment

History

Distinguish between loss of acuity, field, brightness, contrast, and colour. Enquire specifically for diplopia, and if present whether it is horizontal or has a vertical component, and whether it is present in all positions or worse in any direction. Distinguish diplopia from oscillopsia.

Establish as far as possible the duration and variability of symptoms, bearing in mind that uniocular visual loss may go unnoticed by the patient for a long time and falsely thought to be recent, and that diplopia and oscillopsia are always of sudden onset.

Examination

Measure the visual acuities, uncorrected and best-corrected. Examine the pupils for equality of size and relative afferent pupil defect (RAPD). Measure the visual fields, using a technique which is appropriate to the patient and the condition under investigation. Assess red desaturation by comparing the colour percept of a red target of the two eyes individually in turn, and assess colour vision using pseudoisochromatic plates, or the Farnsworth Munsell 100-hue test, as appropriate in the circumstances.

Examine ocular motility, by assessing the movement of both eyes together (conjugate *versions* and dysjugate *vergences*), and individually (*ductions*). Watch slow and fast eye movements, respectively, to a followed and a refixated target, toward the six cardinal positions of gaze and midline elevation and depression. Perform a cover test in eccentric gaze positions if there is diplopia during a version, to reveal muscle paresis. The cardinal positions of gaze are those in which one extraocular muscle is acting maximally while the other five act minimally; diplopia in any cardinal position therefore indicates which muscle action is compromised (see Chapter 9).

Look carefully for nystagmus, and record its vectors. Check the upper lids for ptosis or lagophthalmos.

Examine function in neural pathways anatomically adjacent to a suspected lesion, particularly V, VII, and VIII.

Carry out a complete eye examination, with particular reference to the optic discs, to exclude ocular pathology.

Investigation

Visual fields (Figs 8.1–8.8)

The visual field is that part of space in which objects are visible at the same time during steady fixation. Visual field measurement shows the distribution of threshold across the field, and reveals areas of reduced sensitivity. Lesions at different levels in the visual pathway give rise to patterns of field loss which are characteristic of that level, determined by the anatomical arrangement of nerve fibres. Bear these patterns in mind, and concentrate on vulnerable areas of the field (e.g. the vertical midline), when assessing neurological fields. The various methods of field measurement (see Chapter 1, p. 4) identify threshold of visibility of stimuli at various points across the field. Points with the same

Figs 8.1–8.8: Visual fields

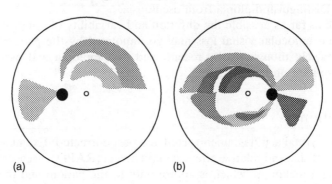

(a)   (b)

Fig. 8.1   (a) Left early glaucoma; (b) right established glaucoma.

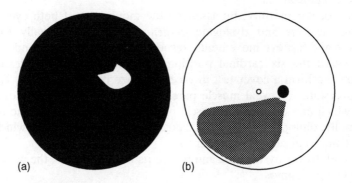

(a)   (b)

Fig. 8.2   (a) Left advanced glaucoma; (b) field in right upper temporal branch retinal vein occlusion, sparing the macula.

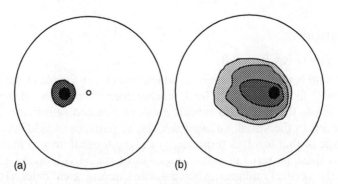

(a)   (b)

Fig. 8.3   (a) Left enlarged blind spot (papilloedema); (b) right centrocaecal scotoma (toxic optic neuropathy).

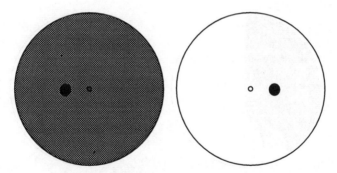

Fig. 8.4 Left eye/optic nerve blindness.

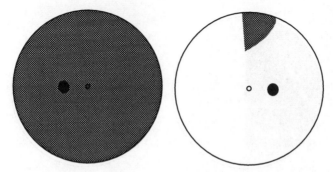

Fig. 8.5 'Junctional' lesion (anterior chiasm) involving left optic nerve and upper temporal field of right eye.

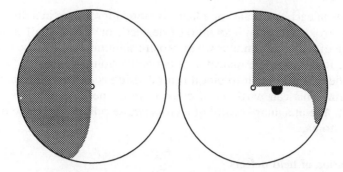

Fig. 8.6 Bitemporal hemianopia, lesion affecting chiasm.

threshold are joined to show lines of equal sensitivity, called isopters. The projection of the fovea is the centre of the visual field.

Choose a perimetric technique which is appropriate to the circumstances: management of chiasmal compression or identification of a centrocaecal defect requires meticulous and sensitive recording (Goldman or computerized perimeters, or Bjerrum screen), but confrontation testing to hand or finger

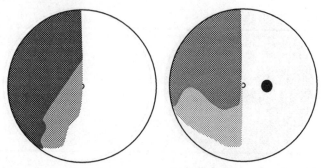

Fig. 8.7 Incongruous left homonymous hemianopia, lesion affecting right optic radiation.

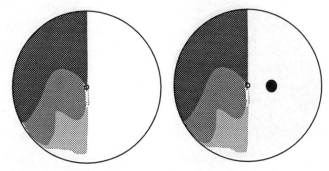

Fig. 8.8 Congruous left homonymous hemianopia, lesion affecting right occipital cortex.

movements in each quadrant, or a light, is more appropriate in a drowsy patient following stroke. Sensory inattention ('neglect', or 'extinction') describes the perception of only one stimulus when two are simultaneously presented, one on each side. It is a sensitive indicator of parietal lesions.

Visual fields are difficult to plot if central vision is impaired, because fixation is uncertain. This can partly be overcome, in cooperative subjects, by having them fixate the imaginary centre of a cross whose points are visible outside the central scotoma.

Interpretation of field defects

1. Uniocular defects are caused by pre-chiasmal pathology. (Fig. 8.4)
2. If there is a uniocular defect, always look carefully for a junctional (upper temporal) scotoma in the other eye ('pie in the sky'), indicating a lesion which includes the anterior chiasm. (Fig. 8.5)
3. Chiasmic or postchiasmic disorder produces a defect which respects the vertical midline. (Figs 8.5–8.8)
4. Nasal field defects due to glaucoma respect the horizontal midline ('nasal step'). (Fig. 8.1)

5. Bitemporal defects indicate chiasmic pathology. (Fig. 8.6)
6. Homonymous defects indicate postchiasmic pathology. (Figs 8.7–8.8)
7. The more congruity (i.e. similarity) between right and left fields in a homonymous hemianopia, the closer the lesion is to the occipital cortex. (Figs 8.7–8.8)
8. Retinal vascular lesions produce a field defect whose apex is at the blind spot, not the visual fixation centre. (Fig. 8.2b)
9. Disc anomalies (e.g. tilted disc) often produce field abnormalities which mimic neurological defects by appearing to be hemianopic. Careful plotting shows that they do not respect the true vertical midline.

Radiological imaging

Since CT has become widely available the indications for plain radiographs of the skull and angiography in neuro-ophthalmological diagnosis have become fewer. It is wise to discuss problems in clinical diagnosis with radiological colleagues, in order that the most appropriate investigations can be undertaken. CT generally gives substantially more clinical information than even the most useful plain film, and will usually be required whatever the latter shows. For example, in the investigation of suspected pituitary tumour, if a plain film shows erosion of the sella, CT will be required to assess the extent of the tumour; negative plain film findings exclude a pituitary tumour with less certainty than a normal CT.

Electrodiagnosis

Visual evoked response (VER)

VER is a sensitive test of function in the optic nerve and geniculostriate projection. The latency between a pattern reversal stimulus presented to one eye and the first positive wave recorded from an occipital scalp electrode (P1) is normally less than 120 ms; a longer delay interval indicates slowed optic nerve conduction, generally due to demyelination. Reduced VER amplitude requires more cautious interpretation, as this may be influenced by both technical and psychological as well as pathological factors. Uniocular VER response may be reduced in compressive and ischaemic optic nerve disease. VER is also useful in the diagnosis of cortical disease (e.g. occipital lobe infarct).

VER is also useful in the assessment of vision in infants. When visual function is in doubt, a normal VER response is an encouraging indication of function in retina, optic nerves, and cortex (although it is not truly direct evidence of visual function).

Electroretinogram (ERG) and electro-oculogram (EOG)

The principal value of these investigations is in the diagnosis of inherited ocular disorders. Attenuated or absent ERG response to a flicker stimulus in photopic illumination indicates primary cone dysfunction, while reduced scotopic ERG implies rod dysfunction. EOG is often impaired early in the course of pigmentary retinopathy; the changes may coincide with nyctalopia, and precede clinical fundus abnormalities.

The visual sensory system

Retinal disorders

The macula and papillomacular bundle are damaged in degenerative, inflammatory, metabolic, toxic, and drug-induced disorders, which are discussed in Chapter 4. The neuro-ophthalmological importance of these conditions lies principally in identifying or excluding an ocular cause for visual loss in the course of neuro-ophthalmological assessment.

In interpreting visual fields it should be remembered that the fovea is at the centre of both the horizontal and vertical midlines, and the blind spot (projection of the disc) is centred some 15°–20° temporal to the centre of the field.

Optic disc and nerve

The aetiology and features of optic neuropathy are summarized in Table 8.1.

Anterior ischaemic optic neuropathy (AION)

Aetiology

- vasculitis, especially giant cell arteritis (GCA),
- hypertension,
- arteriosclerosis.

AION causes a RAPD, with altitudinal field loss, involving central and either upper or lower field.

GCA (temporal) must be confirmed or excluded, as this condition can be treated in order to reduce the risk to the fellow optic nerve, involvement of which may cause complete blindness. GCA seldom occurs in patients below 55 years old, and its incidence increases with age thereafter. Erythrocyte sedimentation rate (ESR) should be measured immediately in all patients presenting with a suspicion of GCA (clinically AION, especially with symptoms of malaise, anorexia, and weight loss, however vague), and artery biopsy arranged if appropriate. The diagnosis is not always straightforward; GCA has been reported in the presence of a normal ESR, and 'skip' segments of normal artery are described. Treatment is with steroids, initially 100 mg hydrocortisone, i.v. or 60–80 mg prednisolone orally, followed by a reducing dose of oral prednisolone, titrated against symptoms and ESR, over 6–24 months.

Papilloedema

The term papilloedema is used to denote disc swelling in association with raised CSF pressure. This is usually due to intracranial CSF obstruction, but if only one disc is involved the cause may be nerve compression.

Table 8.1   Aetiology and features of optic neuropathy

Demyelinating/inflammatory		retrobulbar neuritis	
Vascular (AION)		giant cell arteritis	
		arteriosclerosis, hypertension	
Nutritional		nutritional deficiency	B vitamins (thiamine, B_{12})
Toxic		drugs	ethambutol
			streptomycin
			isoniazid
			chloroquine and hydroxychloroquine
		toxins	tobacco/ethanol
			methanol
			cassava
		heavy metals	
Endocrine		thyroid ophthalmopathy	
Compression	primary	glioma	
		meningioma (nerve sheath, sphenoid ridge)	
	secondary	local spread (nasopharyngeal, pituitary, craniopharyngioma)	
		metastasis	
	benign	Paget's disease	
		sphenoid sinus mucocoele	
Hereditary	Dominant optic atrophy	gradual onset 4–8 years	
		moderate visual loss 6/18–6/60	
		temporal disc pallor	
	Recessive optic atrophy	rare	
		early onset (< 2 years)	
		profound visual failure	
		disc pallor marked	
		associated CNS abnormalities	
	Leber's optic atrophy	affects males usually (mitochondrial inheritance)	
		onset 15–35 years	
		disc and peripapillary small vessel dilatation and telangiectasia	
		bilateral involvement and profound visual loss within months	

Aetiology

Raised intracranial pressure:

- compressive CSF flow obstruction,
- benign intracranial hypertension.

Signs

- Evolving papilloedema   blurred disc margin;

  disc vessel hyperaemia, capillary dilatation, microaneurysms;

  disc margin haemorrhages;

disc swelling/elevation (best seen with 90D lens at slit-lamp);

absent spontaneous disc vessel pulsation (also absent in 20 per cent normal eyes).

- Established papilloedema   peripapillary haemorrhage;

cotton wool spots;

macular 'star' (hand exudates).

Fluorescein angiography shows hyperaemia, vessel leakage from, and late staining of the disc.

The visual field shows enlargement of the blind spot (Fig. 8.3a), as function is compromised in the oedematous peripapillary retinal elements. Associated focal disc lesions (probably caused by localized ischaemic damage) may cause a variety of patterns of concurrent scotoma.

Papilloedema in one disc in the presence of contralateral optic atrophy was originally described (Foster–Kennedy syndrome) as due to a slowly growing frontal tumour, which compressed one nerve having already caused optic atrophy in the other. More commonly the appearance is due to raised intracranial pressure in a patient in whom pre-existing, unrelated pathology had caused prior optic atrophy in one disc (pseudo-Foster–Kennedy)

Optic neuritis

Inflammation affecting the ocular part of the nerve is called papillitis, and abnormal signs are present. Posterior involvement is called retrobulbar neuritis (RBN), and the disc appears to be normal (though fluorescein angiography may show leakage).

Symptoms of optic neuritis

Visual loss

- Decreased uniocular acuity becoming progressively worse over several days.
- May be severe (counting fingers or perception of light).
- Colours are 'washed out' (desaturated), especially red (test for red desaturation by asking the patient to evaluate the 'redness' of a red test object, in turn with the good and then the affected eye).
- The visual deficit usually recovers to some extent over several weeks.

Discomfort

Retrobulbar ache or pain, 'pulling' or 'pricking', especially on extraocular movement, in RBN.

Signs

- *RAPD.*
- *Disc signs*: papillitis presents with disc swelling. In RBN there are no abnormal ophthalmoscopic signs, though fluorescein angiography shows vascular leakage. Disc pallor follows both papillitis and RBN.

Aetiology

Demyelination

- Most common in females aged 20–40 years.
- Approximately 50 per cent have, or will eventually have clinical evidence of multiple sclerosis (MS).
- Up to 80 per cent of patients with clinically isolated RBN have MRI evidence of demyelination elsewhere in the brain.
- 15 per cent of patients with MS begin with RBN.
- MS presenting with RBN has a better prognosis than MS presenting with brainstem signs.

Viral, postviral

In children acute febrile viral illness may precede optic neuropathy, which is often bilateral, and not associated with later development of MS. Optic neuritis associated with Epstein–Barr virus infection has a particularly good prognosis.

Encephalitis

Diagnosis

- The clinical picture is usually sufficient.
- VER latency > 120 ms confirms optic nerve demyelination.

Management

An isolated episode of RBN is self-limiting, and vision recovers to some extent, though there is usually a residual loss of acuity, contrast, brightness, and colour. The possibility that this episode is a part of MS must be borne in mind, and neurological referral should be considered. There is little reason to alarm the patient by discussing the possibility of MS at the first attack.

Treatment with systemic steroids may shorten the course of a demyelinating episode, but has no effect on the final visual acuity.

Congenital disc abnormalities

The disc may appear 'tilted', entering the eye obliquely, in association with an anomalous vessel arrangement. Field defects resembling hemianopia, but which do not respect the true (neurological) transcentral midline, are common in congenitally tilted discs. They are non-progressive and their principal importance lies in their recognition, and the avoidance of unnecessary neuro-ophthalmological investigation.

Optic chiasm

The arrangement of fibres and fields changes from monocular to hemifield at the chiasm, with the result that field abnormalities due to diseases affecting the chiasm are sensitive to the vertical midline. The chiasm is not vulnerable to ischaemia, because of its rich blood supply, which is derived from the internal carotid, anterior and middle cerebral, and posterior communicating arteries. Chiasm pathology is most commonly due to compression (Table 8.2), and its relations are therefore important (Table 8.3).

The precise relation between the chiasm and pituitary is rather variable, the posterior part of a 'prefixed' chiasm being related to the sella, whereas a 'post-fixed' chiasm lies above the pituitary stalk, with only its anterior fibers above the pituitary.

Tumours arising from midline structures characteristically damage the crossing nasal fibres, producing bitemporal hemianopia (Fig. 8.6). This is often not symmetrical, but a true hemianopic pattern can always be demonstrated by a drop in sensitivity precisely across the vertical midline. This sign can be shown by confrontation with a red pin, or more formally using Goldman perimetry. Variations in field loss caused by pituitary tumour depend on the relative positions of the chiasm and pituitary:

1. *Anterior* lesions cause field loss which is mainly monocular, with variable upper temporal loss in the other eye. A loop of inferonasal fibres (the anterior knee of Wilbrand) crosses into the opposite optic nerve before entering the chiasm. These fibres are involved in anterior chiasm lesions, producing an isolated junctional scotoma ('pie in the sky', Fig. 8.5) in the upper temporal field of the other eye. Look carefully for a junctional scotoma in uniocular visual loss which may be caused by a mass involving the chiasm.

Table 8.2   Causes of chiasm compression

Tumour	pituitary
	suprasellar meningioma
	craniopharyngioma
	nasopharyngeal carcinoma
	glioma
	secondary
Aneurysm	internal carotid
	anterior cerebral
	anterior communicating

Table 8.3   Relations of the chiasm

Posterior	III ventricle
	hypothalamus
	pituitary stalk
Inferior	sphenoid
	pituitary gland
Superior	anterior cerebral artery
	anterior communicating artery
	III ventricle (optic recess)
	lamina terminalis of diencephalon
Lateral	internal carotid artery

2. *Central* chiasmic lesions involve the temporal fields of both eyes more or less equally.
3. *Posterior* lesions become increasingly homonymous (the defect involves the same side in the fields of both eyes) towards the optic tracts.

Optic tract, radiation, and cortex

Disease affecting the posterior visual pathway is most commonly vascular, or due to compression by tumour.

Postchiasmal field defects are homonymous hemianopic (Fig. 8.7). They become increasingly congruous (i.e. nearly identical) towards the cortex. Cortical lesions are precisely congruous (Fig. 8.8).

The tracts leave the chiasm, and pass posteriorly around the cerebral peduncles to reach the lateral geniculate nuclei, where they synapse. From the LGN the pathway continues as the optic radiations in the deep temporal and parietal lobes to the occipital pole, where they terminate in the occipital cortex. Fibres in the optic radiation have increasingly accurate binocular registration, accounting for the increasing congruity of posterior lesions.

The visual centre (fixation) may be selectively spared in vascular cortical lesions, probably because its location on the cortex is supplied by both the middle cerebral and posterior cerebral circulation. An area of cortex supplied by one arterial source may therefore infarct, while the macular projection is spared by its dual supply from the internal carotid and basilar circulations.

Lesions involving secondary and associative parts of the visual cortex produce visual disorders more complex than field loss, including hallucination and visual agnosia.

The oculomotor system

Movement of the two eyes in the same direction is called a *conjugate* gaze deviation; movement of the eyes in opposite directions is *dysjugate*. Conjugate movements are described as *versions*, and dysjugate movements as *vergences* (convergence and divergence). *Duction* refers to the movement of one eye.

Versions are driven from the gaze centres in the paramedian pontine reticular formation (PPRF), which are themselves controlled by the frontal and occipital cortex, the vestibular system and the cerebellum. Vergence movements arise in the mid-brain reticular formation. Both these control centres feed into the oculomotor nuclei, to produce appropriate muscle actions via III, IV, and VI nerves.

The control of eye movements (Fig. 8.9)

Supranuclear

Eye movements are generated in response to inputs from the frontal cortex (voluntary), occipital cortex (visually monitored), and cerebellum (eye and head

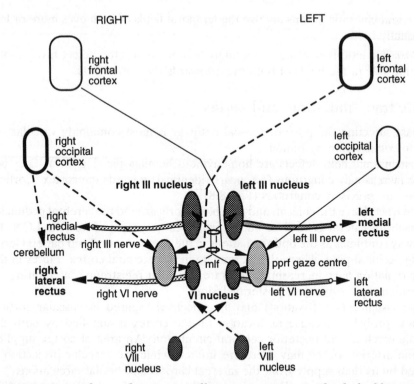

Fig. 8.9 Supranuclear pathways controlling eye movements. The dashed lines show the pathways serving right gaze-deviation, driven by left frontal cortex (frontal eye field, driving saccade) and right occipital cortex (driving pursuit). Note the MLF connection from right VI nucleus to left III nucleus, yoking right lateral rectus with left medial rectus to produce right gaze-deviation.

position). These are integrated with vestibular input in the brainstem gaze centres. The gaze centres project to the ocular motor nuclei, giving rise to a pattern of discharge in III, IV, and VI which produces a conjugate deviation of gaze.

Supranuclear eye movement organization produces two classes of eye movement: slow (SEM) and fast (FEM). SEM are visually controlled and driven by the ipsilateral visual cortex. They are exemplified by the *smooth pursuit* of a target moved across the visual field, and the steady fixation of a stationary target during movement of the head. FEMs are responsible for refixating a new target; vision is suppressed during an FEM, and the path of the eyes is 'ballistic' (i.e. it is pre-programmed before the movement begins). A voluntary refixating FEM is called a *saccade*. Saccades are driven from the frontal eye field of the contra-lateral prefrontal motor cortex.

FEMs can be either voluntary or reflex; all SEMs necessarily have a reflex component, which co-ordinates the position of the eyes in the orbits with the visual field.

Vertical gaze is bilaterally represented at cortical level, projecting to midbrain vertical gaze centres. Vertical eye movement disorder usually indicates midbrain pathology.

Nuclear

Supranuclear input from the gaze centres determines the pattern of discharge from the nuclei to the extraocular muscles.

The gaze centres project to the ipsilateral VI nucleus, to produce abduction in the ipsilateral eye. An interneurone crosses in the medial longitudinal fasciculus (MLF) to the contralateral III nucleus. Corresponding discharge in III causes contraction in the contralateral medial rectus, and adduction in that eye. In this way the movements of the two eyes are yoked, to produce versions, or conjugate gaze deviations.

Extraocular muscle stimulation is combined with inhibition of the ipsilateral antagonist (Sherrington's law), to produce smooth eye movement. The two muscles which produce movement of the two eyes in a given direction (e.g. left lateral rectus and right medial rectus in left gaze) are called a yoke pair. The two muscles of a yoke pair receive equal innervation (Hering's law).

Infranuclear

In the orbit, III divides into a superior division, which innervates superior rectus and levator, and an inferior division which innervates medial and inferior rectus and inferior oblique. VI innervates lateral rectus and IV innervates superior oblique.

Lesions affecting the motor nerves produce uniocular motility disorder, causing paralytic squint and diplopia. The affected nerve can be identified from the pattern of paresis (see Chapter 9).

Lesions of the motor nerves occur in the brainstem (nucleus and fasciculus), along their intracranial course, or in the cavernous sinus or the orbital apex. Their causes are summarized in Tables 8.6–8.8.

Testing supranuclear eye movements

Voluntary eye movements

Saccade

Alternate fixation and refixation between two targets, to either side of, and above and below, central fixation.

Pursuit

Instruct the patient to follow a target moved slowly across the field from one side to the other, and back. Watch carefully for instability or jerkiness of the eyes' pursuit movement.

Normal voluntary saccades and pursuits indicate that the frontal and occipital cortex, and their descending pathways through the brainstem nuclei to the extraocular muscles, are functionally intact. If there is a defect of voluntary conjugate gaze, test the response to reflex stimulation (Table 8.4). Defective voluntary

Table 8.4   Tests of reflex eye movement

Doll's head
Movement of the eyes opposite to the direction of a brisk horizontal or vertical passive head movement. Afferent from vestibular nuclei.

Caloric stimulation
Tonic deviation of the eyes towards (or nystagmus away from) the side of a labyrinth stimulated by cold water syringed into the external auditory meatus. Afferent from vestibular nuclei.

Bell's phenomenon
Upward deviation of the eyes on active lid closure. Arises in mid-brain.

saccades but intact reflex deviation indicates a cortical or mid-brain lesion; if both voluntary and reflex gaze are defective, the lesion is in the brainstem gaze centre.

Reflex eye movements

Optokinetic nystagmus (OKN)

Rotate an optokinetic drum (or pass an OKN tape) towards first one side, and then the other. A defective optokinetic nystagmus response towards one side indicates frontal, parietal, or occipital lesion on that side. The OKN response comprises SEMs (derived from the ipsilateral occipital cortex, passing through the deep parietal cortex) in the direction of movement of the drum stripes, and refixating FEMs (driven by the frontal cortex on the same side) toward the opposite direction. Thus a hemisphere lesion affects each component of OKN.

OKN testing reveals lesions which may not be evident on testing the response to simple saccades and pursuits.

Vestibulo-ocular reflex (VOR)

The VOR is the basis of the eyes' response to rotation, maintaining a constant relation between eye position and field during head movements. It can be tested by rotation in a Barany chair, or more conveniently by the 'doll's head' manoeuvre. Rotate briskly (but gently) the head of a patient who cannot make voluntary eye movements, to one side and then the other, through an excursion of 15°–20°. If the VOR is normal the eyes will rotate in the orbits, remaining fixed on a stationary target ahead in spite of the head movement. If the eyes remain still in the orbits, VOR is defective.

Caloric tests

Warm water irrigating the external auditory meatus causes a sustained gaze deviation away from the irrigated side, or nystagmus with its fast phase directed towards the irrigated side. Cold water irrigation causes opposite deviations. Caloric tests are useful in evaluating the neurological status of comatose patients.

If voluntary eye movements are defective but reflexes are intact, the lesion is cortical. If both voluntary and reflex movements are defective, the lesion is either in the brainstem, or due to ocular myopathy.

Supranuclear eye movement disorders

Horizontal movements

Lesions of the frontal cortex (frontal eye field) affect saccades. They may be irritative acutely, causing sustained unsteady gaze deviation to the opposite side, but become paralytic within a week or two, causing sustained deviation towards the side of the lesion (due to unopposed action in the opposite, normal, frontal eye field).

Lesions of the occipital cortex impair visually guided pursuit, causing failure of smooth pursuit towards the side of the lesion and OKN asymmetry. Sparing of reflex gaze deviations distinguishes cortical from brainstem lesions.

Brainstem lesions involving the gaze centres in the PPRF affect both voluntary and reflex gaze deviations. Ipsilateral movement is paralysed, causing sustained gaze deviation away from the side of the lesion, which cannot be overcome by command, pursuit or reflex stimulation.

Vertical movements

Vertical movements have bilateral cortical representation, and are driven by vertical gaze centres in the mid-brain. This centre is affected in the dorsal mid-brain (Parinaud's) syndrome (elevation palsy, convergence retraction nystagmus, and dilated, light-near dissociated pupils).

Combined horizontal and vertical movements

Steele–Richardson syndrome (pseudo-ophthalmoplegia, or progressive supranuclear palsy), is produced by generalized degeneration in the basal ganglia and mid-brain. It affects (initially by slowing) saccades before pursuits, and vertical gaze before horizontal gaze. There are extrapyramidal parkinsonian features, and truncal rigidity in extension. Reflex eye movements are preserved initially, but as the degenerative process extends down the brainstem, these too may be lost.

Nuclear and infranuclear eye movement disorders

Lesions involving the nuclei of III, IV, or VI in the brainstem produce uniocular paresis of the eye movement driven by that nerve. IV crosses the dorsal brainstem in the superior medullary velum, so that the IV nuclei innervate the contralateral eye; all others innervate ipsilaterally. Nuclear III and VI lesions generally involve adjacent brainstem nuclei and pathways (Table 8.5).

The motor nerves may be damaged in their intracerebral (Table 8.6), intracranial (Table 8.7), or intracavernous parts, or in the superior orbital fissure (Table 8.8). Aetiological factors may be general or specific.

Table 8.5   Syndromes associated with nuclear and fascicular lesions of III and VI

	Structures		Signs
III	red nucleus	Benedikt's	contralateral extrapyramidal signs
	corticospinal tract	Weber's	contralateral upper motor neurone paresis
VI	gaze centre		paresis of ipsilateral conjugate gaze involving willed and reflex deviations
	gaze centre, V, VII, and VIII nucleus	Foville's	gaze paresis, ipsilateral hemifacial paresis and paraesthesia, and ipsilateral hearing loss
	Foville's + pyramidal	Millard–Gubler	Foville's + contralateral hemiparesis
	MLF and VI nucleus		internuclear ophthalmoplegia and abduction paresis

Identify infranuclear disorder (motor nerve paresis or muscle palsy) by testing ductions in the six cardinal positions of gaze, as described in Chapter 9, p. 171.

Ocular motor defects can also have causes other than focal neurological lesions (Table 8.9).

Intracerebral lesions

Nuclear and fascicular lesions (Table 8.6) usually involve adjacent nuclei and pathways (Table 8.5).

Intracranial lesions (Table 8.7)

III

Pupil-sparing ('external') III involves only fibres to the extraocular muscles and levator. It presents as diplopia without unequal pupils, and its aetiology is

Table 8.6   Aetiology of intracerebral ocular motor nerve lesions

Vascular	ischaemic
	haemorrhagic
Aneurysm	
Neoplastic	primary
	secondary
Demyelination	
Infective	meningitis, encephalitis
	abscess
	cyst

Table 8.7 Some causes of intracranial lesions of ocular motor nerves

Nerve	Cause	
General	vascular	diabetes
		hypertension
		arteriosclerosis
		vasculitis (giant cell arteritis, SLE, PAN)
	tumour	primary
		secondary
	aneurysm	
	inflammatory	meningitis
		encephalitis
		Miller–Fisher syndrome
		herpes zoster
	demyelination	
	trauma	
	ophthalmoplegic migraine	
III	aneurysm	posterior communicating
		posterior cerebral
		basilar
		intracavernous internal carotid artery
	tumour	
	trauma	
IV	congenital	
	trauma	avulsion at exit from dorsal mid-brain
		often bilateral
	herpes zoster	
VI	raised intracranial pressure	head injury
		intracranial inflammation
		intracranial haemorrhage
		tumour
	aneurysm	ant inf cerebellar
		post inf cerebellar
		basilar
		internal carotid (in cavernous sinus)
	Gradenigo's syndrome	VI involvement in petrous inflammation, in otitis media
	Cerebellopontine angle tumour	

generally vascular ('medical III'). The pupil fibres lie externally in the nerve, are supplied by pial vessels, and are therefore spared in occlusion of vasa nervorum. Vascular III palsy is managed conservatively, with Fresnel prisms or occlusion to relieve diplopia, and usually resolves in 6–12 weeks.

Diabetes and arteriosclerosis are the commonest causes of 'vascular' III palsy.

Complete ('surgical') III involves the pupil as well as the extraocular muscles. It presents with exotropia and ptosis and a dilated pupil on the affected side. It

Table 8.8 Aetiology of lesions of ocular motor nerves in the cavernous sinus and SOF

Aneurysm		
Caroticocavernous fistula		
Tumour	parasellar extension of pituitary tumour	
	craniopharyngioma	
	nasopharyngeal carcinoma	
	metastasis	
Cavernous sinus thrombosis		
Herpes zoster		
Lymphoma		
Pseudotumour and Tolosa–Hunt		
Sphenoid sinus mucocoele		

Table 8.9 Ocular motility disorder without a focal neurological lesion

Dysthyroid eye disease		
Myasthenia gravis		
Decompensated heterophoria		
Congenital	Duane's lid-retraction syndrome	
	Moebius	
Ocular myopathy		
Post-traumatic or postsurgical restrictive myopathy		

is usually due to compressive pathology (aneurysm or tumour). Urgent surgical intervention may be necessary; acute pupil-involving III palsy requires full neurological examination and CT scan without delay.

Both medical (vascular) and surgical III may be painful or painless.

IV

IV decussates on the dorsal surface of the brainstem, taking a long course between the posterior cerebral and superior cerebellar arteries to enter the lateral wall of the cavernous sinus. It is vulnerable to aneurysm and injury. Acceleration–deceleration injuries commonly cause bilateral avulsion of the nerves as they leave the brainstem.

Zoster frequently involves IV in its intracranial course, causing vertical diplopia.

VI

VI leaves the inferior pons to climb over the edge of the petrous temporal bone and enter the cavernous sinus. It may be damaged by cerebral oedema due to raised intracranial pressure (caused by trauma, tumour, or inflammation) as it crosses the petrous bone. It is also characteristically involved in tumours of the cerebellopontine angle (with loss of corneal sensation and hearing loss), and severe otitis media. Corneal sensation and hearing should always be tested, and the optic discs inspected for papilloedema, in VI palsy.

Vascular VI lesions are common in the elderly and arteriopaths. These are managed conservatively, with Fresnel prisms and serial Hess charts, and usually begin to resolve within 6 weeks. Like vascular III, they may be painful or painless. VI palsy which fails to recover spontaneously requires transposition surgery (Jensen's or Hummelsheim procedure) to relieve the diplopia.

Nerve lesions in the cavernous sinus (Fig. 8.10).

III (and the parasympathetics), IV, V_1, and V_2, and the sympathetics, pass through the dura forming the lateral wall of the cavernous sinus; VI runs free within the sinus.

Pathology in the cavernous sinus (Table 8.7) affects some or all of these nerves, VI being the most vulnerable and earliest affected. The clinical picture is of a painful progressive ophthalmoplegia, with periorbital sensory disturbance, and variable vascular engorgement.

Nerve lesions in the superior orbital fissure and orbital apex (Fig. 8.11)

The nerves leaving the cavernous sinus enter the orbit through the superior orbital fissure. The optic nerve enters the orbit separately, with the sympathetics, through the optic canal. Orbital apex pathology presents with ophthalmoplegia, pain, and variable proptosis; simultaneous involvement of the optic foramen is indicated by visual loss, relative afferent pupil defect (RAPD), and optic disc signs. Orbital apex disease is most commonly due to chronic lymphocytic inflammation; anterior extension of a sphenoid ridge meningioma, and orbital lymphoma, may present with a similar clinical picture.

Orbital disease

Focal involvement of the ocular motor nerves in the orbit is uncommon. Ocular motility disorder caused by orbital pathology is usually due to involvement of

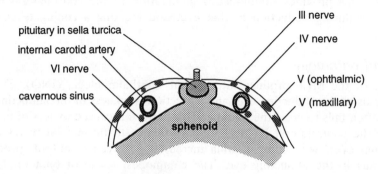

Fig. 8.10   The structures passing through the cavernous sinus. VI is free within the sinus, and is especially vulnerable to damage by internal carotid artery aneurysm. III, IV, V_1, and V_2 travel in the dural wall of the sinus.

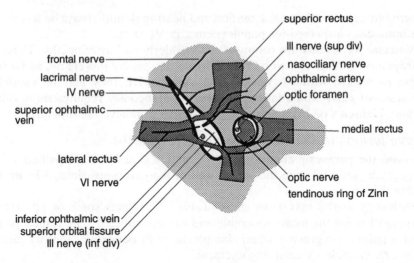

Fig. 8.11 The apex of the orbit. All structures except the optic nerve, ophthalmic artery and sympathetics enter through the superior orbital fissure. All extraocular muscle nerves except IV pass through the tendinous ring of Zinn.

the extraocular muscles by inflammation, trauma, or tumour, causing mechanical restriction or local paresis, or to myasthenia.

Internuclear ophthalmoplegia

Anatomy (Fig. 8.9)
The gaze centres in the PPRF project to the ipsilateral VI nucleus. Motor cells in this nucleus send axons in the VI nerve to the lateral rectus, producing ipsilateral abduction, and collateral axons in the MLF to the contralateral III nucleus. This provides simultaneous innervation to the contralateral medial rectus, producing adduction in that eye, and creating a conjugate gaze deviation.

Clinical pathology
Lesions of the MLF produce internuclear ophthalmoplegia (INO). There is nystagmus of the abducting eye, and adduction weakness in the adducting eye, which often fails to cross the midline. This pattern is caused by loss of innervation to the contralateral III nucleus (and thence to the medial rectus of the adducting eye), with compensating increased gaze centre output, producing nystagmus in the abducting eye. The commonest cause of bilateral INO is demyelinating disease, while unilateral INO is most commonly vascular. Myasthenia gravis may produce a similar pattern of movement disorder, though the cause is not central but at the neuromuscular junction.

Nystagmus

Oscillating eye movements indicate instability of the oculomotor control system in the brainstem. The cause of nystagmus can be identified by observation of its pattern: record its direction and intensity (velocity and amplitude of excursion) diagrammatically in the primary and eight eccentric gaze positions, with arrows showing the direction of the fast phase (Figs 8.12–8.15). The thickness of their shafts represents amplitude, and the number of their tails represents frequency. Nystagmus causes visual impairment according to its intensity, and the coexistence of associated disorders.

Classification
- congenital nystagmus (CN),
- vestibular nystagmus (VN),
- gaze-evoked (central) nystagmus (GEN).

Congenital nystagmus (CN) (Fig. 8.12)

CN may occur as an isolated phenomenon, or in association with a specific

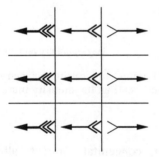

Congenital nystagmus

Fig. 8.12   Congenital nystagmus. The nystagmus is uniplanar horizontal, regardless of direction of gaze, but its frequency and amplitude vary with horizontal gaze deviation. The null point and reversal are to the left of the midline in this example.

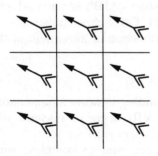

Vestibular nystagmus

Fig. 8.13   Vestibular nystagmus. The nystagmus is multiplanar (mixed horizontal and vertical components), but does not vary with gaze direction.

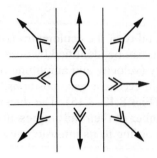

Gaze-evoked nystagmus

Fig. 8.14 Gaze-evoked nystagmus. The nystagmus is directed (fast phase) towards the position of gaze, and is minimal or absent in the primary position.

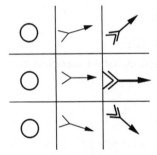

Gaze-paretic nystagmus

Fig. 8.15 Gaze-paretic nystagmus. Following, and during recovery of, paresis of conjugate gaze to the left, nystagmus is left-beating. Its intensity increases with gaze-deviation toward the paretic side.

childhood-onset visual disorder; e.g. congenital cataract; albinism; achromatopsia; Leber's amaurosis.

CN is always uniplanar, and almost always horizontal. The intensity varies with horizontal gaze direction. The gaze position in which the intensity of CN is least, or its direction reverses, is called the null point. Vision is best at the null point, and an abnormal head posture (AHP) is often adopted to exploit this. Oscillopsia is not a feature of CN. OKN characteristically appears to be reversed (i.e. the fast phase is in the direction of movement of the OKN tape or drum) in CN.

Vestibular nystagmus (VN) (Fig. 8.13)

Vestibular nystagmus is acquired, secondary to acute inflammatory, neoplastic or traumatic damage to a labyrinth, VIII nerve or nucleus, which leads to asymmetric vestibular input to the brainstem gaze centres.

It is uniplanar, but may be non-horizontal or complex, with a rotatory element. The direction and intensity are unaffected by gaze-direction. There is oscillopsia and reduction in visual acuity, and other signs of vestibular or VIII disorder (vertigo and tinnitus). Vestibular nystagmus may reduce and resolve as the visual system adjusts to chronic unilateral vestibular disorder.

Reflex vestibular nystagmus and caloric tests

Reflex vestibular nystagmus on rotation, (the VOR), which helps stabilize vision during head movement, is a physiological nystagmus driven by asymmetric input from the vestibular system.

Caloric stimulation of the labyrinths tests reflex eye movements. Cold water stimulates nystagmus with fast beat away from chilled labyrinth; warm irrigation drives fast phase towards the stimulated side (Cold Opposite Warm Same – COWS)

Central or gaze-evoked nystagmus (GEN) (Fig. 8.14)

Central nystagmus is caused by progressive reduction in eye position signal, or 'integrator leak', due to brainstem or cerebellar pathology. The eyes constantly drift back towards the primary from an eccentric gaze position, and this drift is interrupted cyclically by refixating saccades. It is caused by demyelination, tumour, or drugs. The fast beat in GEN is in the direction of gaze, the intensity is maximal on maximal gaze deviation, and nystagmus is minimal or absent in the primary position.

Gaze paretic nystagmus (GPN. Fig. 8.15) is a special form of GEN, occurring in, and during recovery from, unilateral gaze paresis. The fast beat is directed towards the direction of the gaze paresis, maximum on gaze toward the affected side, and minimal or absent in opposite gaze.

Oscillopsia is a feature of GEN, and causes reduced visual acuity.

The autonomic system

The pupil (Fig. 8.16)

The pupil size is determined by the balance between the activity of the sphincter (circular fibres, parasympathetic innervation) and the dilator (radial fibres, sympathetic innervation) muscles. The sphincter can also be stimulated by miotics, which act either directly on the muscle's postsynaptic receptors (pilocarpine), or indirectly, by potentiating the effect of acetylcholine (cholinesterase inhibitors, e.g. physostigmine).

Pupil innervation

The preganglionic *parasympathetic* nerve cell bodies are in the Edinger–Westphal subnucleus of III in the brainstem. They pass in the III nerve intracranially and through the cavernous sinus to enter the orbit through the superior orbital fissure. In the orbit they leave III (branch to inferior oblique), forming the short motor root of the ciliary ganglion, to synapse in the ganglion. Postganglionic fibres enter the eye in short ciliary nerves, to supply the smooth muscles of the iris sphincter and ciliary body.

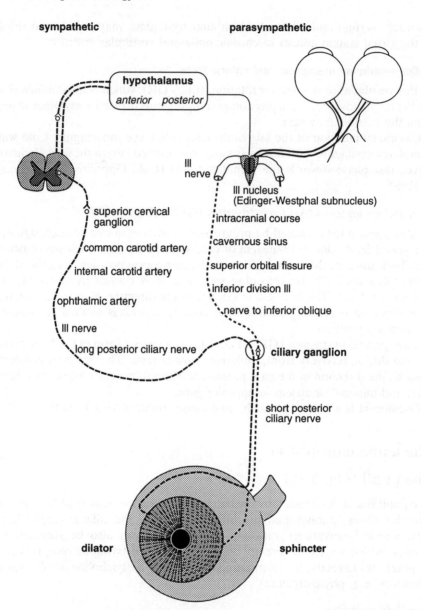

sympathetic   **parasympathetic**

hypothalamus
anterior   posterior

III
nerve

III nucleus
(Edinger-Westphal subnucleus)

superior cervical
ganglion

intracranial course

common carotid artery

cavernous sinus

internal carotid artery

superior orbital fissure

ophthalmic artery

inferior division III

III nerve

nerve to inferior oblique

long posterior ciliary nerve

ciliary ganglion

short posterior
ciliary nerve

dilator   **sphincter**

The *sympathetics* are derived from cells in the hypothalamus, whose fibres pass down in the lateral column of the spinal cord to synapse with the lateral horn cells in the lower cervical and upper thoracic segments. Fibres from these cells leave the cord and enter the sympathetic chain (preganglionic), to synapse in the superior cervical ganglion (SCG). The postganglionic sympathetics travel along the internal carotid and ophthalmic artery to enter the orbit through the superior orbital fissure. They pass through the ciliary ganglion without synapsing,

Fig. 8.16 Pupil pathways. First-order sympathetic neurones are located in the anterior hypothalamus, and descend in the lateral columns to synapse with the lateral horn cells. Second-order sympathetics leave the spinal cord and synapse in the superior cervical ganglion. Third-order fibres travel with the internal carotid and its branches to the orbit, passing through the ciliary ganglion without synapsing, to enter the eye in the posterior ciliary nerves. Periocular sudomotor sympathetics travel with the external carotid. Parasympathetic fibres pass from cells in the Edinger–Westphal nucleus of III to the orbit in the superficial part of the III nerve. The Edinger–Westphal nucleus has bilateral visual input (from the optic tracts, via the brachia of the superior colliculi), and tonic input from the hypothalamus. The parasympathetics synpase in the ciliary ganglion, and second order fibres enter the eye, with sympathetics and sensory fibres, as the posterior ciliary nerves.

---

to gain the eye in short ciliary nerves, as vasomotor and pupil dilator efferents. Horner's syndrome (small pupil caused by loss of sympathetic tone) may be caused by lesions affecting the preganglionic or postganglionic fibres.

Sensory fibres from the eye reach the ciliary ganglion (through which they pass without synapsing) in short ciliary nerves. They leave the ganglion in its long sensory root, to join the nasociliary nerve in the orbit, from whence they reach V_1 and the trigeminal ganglion.

Pupil reflex neuroanatomy (Fig. 8.17)

The afferent fibres serving pupil reflexes leave the optic tracts before the lateral geniculate nuclei, in the brachia of the superior colliculi, to reach the pretectal nuclei. They project from each pretectal nucleus to supply both Edinger–Westphal nuclei, from which the iris sphincters of both eyes are innervated symmetrically. Both pupils therefore respond equally to light shone into either, unless there is a motor defect.

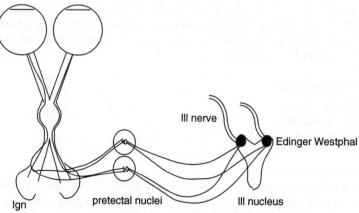

Fig. 8.17 Neuroanatomy of relative afferent pupil defect.

The relative afferent pupil test (RAPD, Marcus–Gunn pupil, swinging flashlight test)

Shine a bright light into each pupil in turn in a regular cycle of 0.5–1 s, and watch the reaction of the pupil of each eye in turn as it is illuminated. The pupil of a normal eye constricts, while the pupil of an eye with optic nerve disease or damage will seem to dilate to the light (because when illuminated it generates less pupil constriction than the normal eye).

The swinging flashlight test is a very important test of differential optic nerve function. It is unaffected by media opacity or macular disease, but is positive only if there is substantially reduced conduction of light information in one optic nerve. This is usually due to optic nerve disease, advanced glaucoma, or retinal detachment. RAPD distinguishes between visual loss which is due to media opacity (e.g. cataract) or maculopathy, and that due to optic nerve or extensive retinal disease.

The afferent pupil test can be carried out even if one pupil is immobile, since both pupils react equally to light shone in either eye, and the pupil reaction of either may be observed.

Anisocoria (unequal pupils)

Anisocoria is caused by a motor pupil defect, and may be due to failure of the smaller pupil to dilate, or failure of the larger pupil to constrict. To distinguish between these, examine the patient in a dark and a light room. If the inequality is greater in darkness, the smaller pupil has failed to dilate, and its dilator (sympathetic) is abnormal. If the inequality is greater in bright illumination, the larger pupil has failed to constrict, and the abnormality is in its sphincter (parasympathetic).

Parasympathetic lesions at, or distal to, the ciliary ganglion produce denervation supersensitivity to direct-acting parasympathomimetic; pilocarpine 0.1 per cent is used to confirm Adie's pupil. Pharmacological pupil tests are described below. They should be performed on eyes which have not been anaesthetized or applanated, since drug absorption by the cornea may be affected. Twenty-four hours should elapse between using cocaine and hydroxyamphetamine in the diagnosis of Horner's syndrome, and weaker concentrations of pilocarpine should be used before stronger.

Causes of a small pupil

- benign anisocoria,
- Horner's syndrome,
- pharmacological.

Benign anisocoria

The pupils are significantly unequal in size in up to 20 per cent of normal eyes without neurological pathology. Their reactions are equal in response to light, dark, and pharmacological stimulation.

Horner's syndrome

Sympathetic lesions deplete the transmitter at the adrenergic synapse, and reduce dilator function. Confirm with one drop of cocaine 4 per cent to each eye: cocaine potentiates noradrenalin (NA) in the synaptic cleft by preventing its reuptake into presynaptic vesicles. If there is a sympathetic lesion, the synaptic cleft has no NA, and Horner's pupil therefore fails to dilate.

Distinguish between preganglionic and postganglionic Horner's using 1 per cent hydroxyamphetamine, which potentiates transmission by displacing NA from the presynaptic vesicles. It therefore dilates a preganglionic Horner's (in which presynaptic vesicles are intact), but fails to dilate a postganglionic Horner's (in which they are depleted, because the postsynaptic nerve ending is isolated from the cell body). The distinction is important, since apical lung malignancy involves preganglionic sympathetics, but postganglionic Horner's are associated with carotid artery, cavernous sinus or orbital apex disease.

Other signs of Horner's syndrome are ptosis (denervation of Müller's muscle) and hypohidrosis over the affected side of the face. Congenital Horner's syndrome causes failure of iris pigmentation, producing heterochromia.

Causes of a large pupil

- complete III nerve palsy,
- Adie's myotonic pupil,
- pharmacological mydriasis,
- traumatic mydriasis.

III nerve palsy

Pupil-involving III nerve lesions are usually compressive. They involve the extraocular muscles (giving rise to exodeviation and depression) as well as the pupils. It is important to exclude pre-existing anisocoria in a patient with III palsy and pupil signs.

Distinguish between the various causes of a large pupil using pilocarpine: measure the pupil diameters at the slit-lamp; put one drop of pilocarpine 0.1 per cent in each eye and measure the pupils again after 15 min; repeat using pilocarpine 1 per cent.

- 0.1 per cent pilocarpine   Adie's pupil constricts (supersensitivity);
                             normal pupils, III palsy, constrict significantly less;
                             pharmacologically dilated pupils do not constrict;
- 1 per cent pilocarpine   Adie's, III palsy, normal pupils constrict;
                             pharmacological pupils do not constrict (parasympathetic blockade).

Adie's myotonic pupil

Adie's is an abnormally dilated pupil, showing spontaneous 'vermiform' movement at its margin, constricting poorly, or not at all, to light, but slowly to prolonged convergence. Accommodation is impaired by simultaneous ciliary muscle weakness. It is sometimes associated with deep tendon hyporeflexia (Holmes–Adie's syndrome), and occurs most commonly in females 20–40 years, lasting several weeks or months. Confirm Adie's pupil using 0.1 per cent pilocarpine, to which the supersensitive pupil responds with more miosis than normal (see pupil tests). The dynamic abnormalities in Adie's pupil are permanent, though the anisocoria reduces with time. The cause is thought to be disorder in the ciliary ganglion, possibly associated with viral inflammation.

Pharmacological mydriasis
Atropine completely blocks the parasympathetic receptors, causing an immobile dilated pupil. Other mydriatics (tropicamide, phenylephrine) permit some miosis to pilocarpine, but less marked and less quickly than the normal pupil.

Traumatic mydriasis
Pupil sphincter rupture causes an irregular dilated pupil without vermiform movement or supersensitivity. The history of trauma usually precludes confusion, but may not be volunteered without direct questioning.

Irregular pupil

Sector atrophy of the iris dilator follows herpes simplex uveitis, causing irregularity which is most marked on dilation, and is associated with depigmentation and transillumination. Sphincter rupture follows blunt trauma or surgery, and sphincter atrophy may follow acute glaucoma. The resulting dilated pupil may be irregular. Pupil irregularity is also caused by posterior synaechiae following anterior uveitis.

Recommended further reading

Burde, R.M., Savino, P.J., and Trobe, J.D. (1992). *Clinical decisions in neuro-ophthalmology*, 2nd edn. Mosby, St Louis.

Farris, B.K. (1991). *The basics of neuro-ophthalmology*. Mosby, St Louis.

Glaser, J.S. (1990). *Neuro-ophthalmology*, 2nd edn. Lippincott, Philadelphia.

Leigh, R.J. and Zee, D.S. (1983). *The neurology of eye movements*, 2nd edn. Davis, Philadelphia.

Miller, N.R. (1985). *Walsh & Hoyt's clinical neuro-ophthalmology*, 4th edn, 3 vols. Williams & Wilkins, Baltimore.

Walsh, T.J. (1991). *Neuro-ophthalmology. Clinical signs and symptoms*, 3rd edn. Lea & Febiger, Philadelphia.

9
Disorders of ocular motility

Acquired ocular motility disorders

The direction of the visual axis of each eye towards a fixation point is co-ordinated by the action of the extraocular muscles. If the target is at a distant point, the visual axes are parallel; they converge towards a near point. Supra-nuclear and internuclear mechanisms maintain ocular alignment, so that corresponding points on the two retinas receive corresponding images of the visual field, which are fused into a single solid percept.

Strabismus (squint) is a failure of the co-ordination of binocular alignment. It leads inevitably to loss of binocular single vision. Fusion of the two images is replaced either by diplopia or suppression of one image. Strabismus may be caused by orbit, muscle, motor nerve, or brainstem pathology.

This chapter concerns the management of acquired strabismus. Squint in childhood is usually associated with defective binocular single vision, often has a familial background, and is frequently associated with refractive error; it is discussed in the chapter on paediatric ophthalmology. Conjugate gaze and other supranuclear disorders and nystagmus are discussed in Chapter 8.

Definitions

Primary position

Gaze straight ahead, with the visual axes parallel (as in fixing at a distant point).

Heterotropia

Manifest deviation, i.e. failure of the visual axes to meet at the fixation point when both eyes are open.

Manifest convergent squint is described as esotropia (ET), and manifest divergent squint as exotropia (XT).

Vertical squint is referred to the higher (hypertropic) eye; thus vertical squint with the right eye higher is right hypertropia = R/L, or R HT.

Heterophoria

Latent deviation, i.e. failure of the visual axes to meet at the fixation point when they are dissociated (e.g. by monocular occlusion).

Latent convergent and divergent squint are, respectively, esophoria and exophoria, abbreviated EP and XP.

Duction

Movement of one eye.

Adduction refers to medially directed horizontal movement, and abduction is laterally directed horizontal movement. Vertical ductions are called elevation and depression, and torsional ductions are called intorsion and extorsion.

Version

Movement of both eyes in the same direction. Lateral versions are called dextroversion (rightward-directed gaze deviation) and laevoversion (leftward-directed gaze deviation).

Vertical gaze deviations are called elevation and depression.

Vergence

Movement of both eyes in opposite directions. Convergence (medially directed movement of both eyes) is a physiological movement used in near fixation. Divergence beyond the primary position has no physiological binocular function.

Concomitant

Constant angle of deviation irrespective of the direction of gaze. Squint in childhood is generally concomitant (unless, unusually, caused by acquired motor nerve or orbit pathology).

Incomitant

Variable angle of squint, according to gaze direction. Paralytic squint is incomitant, but becomes progressively concomitant as the paretic muscle recovers, or as the ocular motor control system adjusts to the paralysis. Secondary adaptations occur in the ipsilateral antagonist, and contralateral synergist and antagonist muscles.

Diplopia (binocular)

The two elements of binocular double vision which occur in strabismus are:

1. *Confusion.* Images of two different parts of the visual field are perceived simultaneously by central vision.
2. *Diplopia.* A single object is perceived as being located in two different parts of the field (central and peripheral), because its image falls on the fovea of one eye, and a peripheral retinal point of the other eye.

Cover test

Occlusion of one eye to produce dissociation, revealing:

1. *Heterotropia:* movement of the unoccluded eye to take up fixation.
2. *Heterophoria:* movement of the occluded eye under cover away from fixation.

The cover test is described further in Chapter 10. When examining a paralytic squint, perform cover testing in the cardinal positions of gaze in order to identify the paretic muscle.

Anatomy of the eye muscles

The extraocular muscles rotate the eyes about three axes to produce vertical (elevation and depression), horizontal (adduction and abduction), and rotational (intorsion and extorsion) movements. The horizontal recti produce purely horizontal movements; the vertical recti and the obliques have vertical, rotational, and horizontal actions. Their principal effect depends upon the horizontal position of the eye in the orbit, and therefore varies with gaze position.

The geometry of the orbits is shown in Fig. 9.1. All four recti and superior oblique have their origin at the apex of the orbit, while inferior oblique has its origin at the nasal end of the anterior orbital floor. The recti insert anterior to the equator, at 7.5 mm (superior), 7.0 mm (lateral), 6.5 mm (inferior), and 5.5 mm (medial) behind the limbus. The obliques insert behind the equator: the insertion of the superior oblique tendon lies along the lateral border of superior rectus, having been reflected through the pulley of the trochlea at the anterior nasal orbital roof, and the insertion of inferior oblique lies external to the macula. The superior oblique tendon passes beneath the superior rectus, and the inferior oblique passes beneath the inferior rectus. The vertical recti are aligned with the geometric axis of the eye when it is in 23° of abduction (Fig. 9.2). In this position the vertical recti are pure elevators and depressors. In the primary position, and in adduction, the recti also have a ('secondary') torsional action (Fig. 9.3). Similarly the line of action of the obliques would coincide with the axis of the eye in 52° of adduction, where their action would be purely

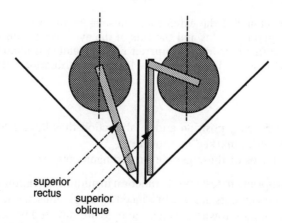

superior
rectus
superior
oblique

Fig. 9.1 The anatomy of the extraocular muscles in the orbits. In the primary position neither vertical recti nor obliques are aligned with the eyes' anatomical axes, and both have mixed vertical, torsional, and horizontal action.

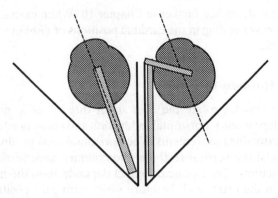

Fig. 9.2 The anatomy of the extraocular muscles in the orbits. In abduction superior rectus is aligned with the eye's anatomical axis, and acts as a pure elevator. In adduction superior oblique tendon is most nearly aligned with the eye's anatomical axis, and the muscle acts mainly as a depressor.

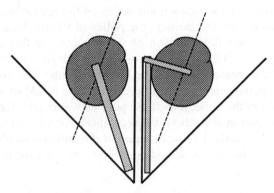

Fig. 9.3 The anatomy of the extraocular muscles in the orbits. In adduction the angle between superior rectus and the axis of the eye gives it intorsional, but little elevating, action. In abduction the superior oblique tendon is almost perpendicular to the eye's anatomical axis, and the muscle acts as an intortor, without depressing action.

vertical. In the primary position and in abduction they have a torsional action, which becomes more marked in abduction.

The consequences of these geometric arrangements are:

1. It is not appropriate to test muscle function in midline elevation and depression, since these movements are not produced by single muscles acting alone. The six positions of gaze towards which the eyes are directed by one muscle each, acting (most nearly) alone, are called the cardinal positions of gaze (Fig. 9.4). Muscle paresis is identified by testing eye movements to these six cardinal positions.

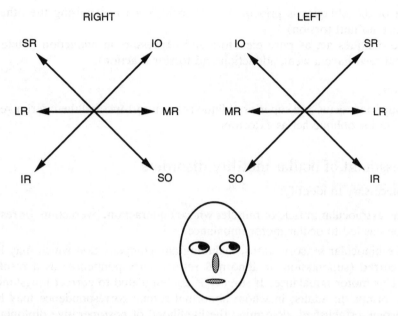

Fig. 9.4 The six cardinal positions of gaze, illustrating the muscle which is principally responsible for each movement, in each eye. The example shows laevoelevation, by left SR and right IO.

2. The vertical recti are tested in abduction. Here they have no rotational action, and the obliques have practically no vertical action.

3. The obliques are tested in adduction. Here their vertical action is greatest and their rotational action least, and it is the position in which the vertical recti contribute least vertical action.

4. In the primary position both superior muscles (SR and SO) are intorters, and the inferior muscles (IR and IO) are extorters.

5. Weakness of an oblique produces vertical or torsional deviation which is maximal when the affected eye is in adduction.

6. Weakness of a vertical rectus produces vertical deviation which is maximal when the affected eye is in abduction.

Eye movements

Horizontal ductions

The horizontal recti are mainly responsible for adduction and abduction. In the primary position the obliques have a small abducting action, and the vertical recti are weak adductors.

Vertical ductions

The vertical recti act as pure elevators and depressors in abduction (while the effect of the obliques is principally rotational, each neutralizing the other to produce no nett torsion).

The obliques act as pure elevators and depressors in adduction (while the vertical recti have a weak adduction and torsional action).

Torsion

The superior rectus and superior oblique act as intortors, and the inferior rectus and inferior oblique act as extortors.

Assessment of ocular motility disorders

It is necessary to identify:

1. The extraocular muscle or muscles whose underaction, overaction, or restriction has led to ocular motor imbalance.
2. The binocular sensory status, including any compensation which may have occurred (suppression or abnormal retinal correspondence) as a result of ocular motor imbalance. If surgery is contemplated to correct longstanding strabismus in adults, in whom abnormal retinal correspondence may have become established, determine the likelihood of postoperative diplopia before operating.

Muscle imbalance

Weakness of any of the 12 extraocular muscles causes diplopia which is maximal in the field of action of that muscle. Two muscles are active in any cardinal position (one for each eye); the paretic muscle is identified by finding the position in which diplopia is maximal, and performing a cover test in this position. The eye seeing the image further from the primary position (the outermost image) has the paretic muscle. This is because an image on the nasal retina is projected to the temporal field, and vice versa.

Muscle imbalance is measured objectively on a Hess (or Lees) screen.

Strabismus of longstanding is compensated by sensory adaptation, replacing diplopia by suppression, or abnormal retinal correspondence.

Binocular vision

Binocular vision describes the quality of simultaneous perception by the two eyes of an object in visual space. In fully developed binocular single vision, fusion of the two slightly different views of an object (caused by the angular separation of the eyes) creates a solid stereoscopic image. This fusion is stable, and can occur over a range of artificially imposed deviations of the visual axes (prism fusion range); less stable grades of binocular function lead to a reduced fusion range. Incompletely developed binocular function may create simultaneous perception with fusion only at the periphery, or simple simultaneous perception without fusion. If binocular function is absent, the image of one eye is suppressed during vision with both eyes open; in childhood the result is amblyopia. Acquired loss of fusion associated with strabismus in later life (due to muscle paresis or restriction, trauma, or cortical disorder) leads to diplopia, which may or may not be compensated by uniocular suppression.

Testing muscle imbalance

Identification of the paretic muscle

Eliminate any abnormal head posture before testing eye movements for muscle imbalance.

Diplopia is maximal in the direction of the field of the paretic muscle; this muscle can quickly be identified in cooperative patients by following a target into the six cardinal positions. In the position of maximal diplopia, determine which of the yoke pair is paretic by cover test. The eye seeing the outermost image has the paretic muscle.

Assess muscle imbalance more formally by determining first whether diplopia is horizontal or vertical; hold a pen vertically and horizontally at a distance of about a metre in the midline. Patients with paresis of a horizontal muscle have purely horizontal diplopia; those with a weak vertical rectus or oblique muscle have a vertical or oblique element to their diplopia.

Horizontal diplopia

The weak muscle must be a horizontal rectus.

1. Is the deviation esotropic or exotropic? Determine whether the diplopia is crossed or uncrossed by occluding one eye and asking whether the right or left image disappears. Uncrossed diplopia (right eye sees right image) occurs in esotropia, and crossed diplopia (right eye sees left image) occurs in exotropia, because of retinal image projection ('eyes crossed = diplopia uncrossed').

2. Which eye has the weak muscle? Assess whether diplopia is greater in left or right gaze. (a) in esotropia: RLR weakness causes greatest diplopia in right gaze; LLR weakness causes greatest diplopia in left gaze. (b) in exotropia: RMR weakness causes greatest diplopia in left gaze; LMR weakness causes greatest diplopia in right gaze.

Vertical diplopia

Paralytic vertical strabismus, causing vertical/oblique diplopia, can be due to paresis or restriction of SR, IR, SO, or IO of either eye, i.e. one of eight muscles. Each is an elevator or a depressor, with a field of vertical action which is maximal either in adduction or abduction. The eight are systematically eliminated to four, two, and finally one possibility using Parks' three-stage test:

1. Determine which is the hypertropic eye. Occlude one eye while a target is fixated, and determine which image is abolished. If the occluded eye had the higher image it is hypotropic, and if it had the lower image it is hypertopic. The weak muscle must be one of the depressors (IR or SO) of the hypertropic eye, or the elevators (SR or IO) of the hypotropic eye: *four possibilities*.

2. Ask the patient to look left and right, and assess in which direction diplopia is maximal. Only one elevator and one depressor act maximally in lateral gaze (the recti in abduction and the obliques in adduction): *two possibilities*.

3. In this position of lateral gaze ask the patient to look up and down. If diplopia is maximal in elevation, the elevator is weak, and if in depression the depressor is weak. Confirm this finding by the Bielschowsky head-tilt test.

The following example illustrates the three-stage test:

1. Identify the higher eye by cover test (eye with lower image). If the right is the higher eye, the failure must be of a: (a) right depressor = *RIR* or *RSO*; or (b) left elevator = *LSR* or *LIO* (four possibilities).

2. The patient fixates a target in left and right gaze. If diplopia is greatest in left gaze, then the affected muscle must be: (a) right depressor = *RSO*; or (b) left elevator = *LSR* (two possibilities).

3. The patient looks left/up (laevoelevation), and left/down (laevodepression). If diplopia is greatest on laevodepression the affected muscle must be *RSO*. Tilt the head to the left and right (Bielschowsky head-tilt test). Head tilt to the right causes elevation of the right eye, as right SR (acting as an intorter) causes simultaneous elevation which is unopposed by right SO.

Bielschowsky head-tilt test

This test confirms superior oblique palsy. Intorsion of the tested eye is provoked by tilting the head towards that side, so that the ear approaches the shoulder, while fixation is maintained in the primary position. SR and SO act as intorters (IR and IO are extorters). If there is a SO weakness on the side of the tilt, the SR intorts alone. Its simultaneous action as elevator is not opposed by SO depression, and the eye is therefore elevated by this manoeuvre, indicating SO weakness.

Abnormal head posture (AHP)

An AHP is an adaptation to minimize the diplopia caused by a paralytic squint. The paretic muscle is unloaded by rotating the affected eye away from its field of action. The head posture is therefore directed towards the field of action of the paretic muscle: e.g. a right lateral rectus palsy results in a right head turn.

AHP is described in terms of:

- horizontal rotation = head turn
- vertical movement = chin up or chin down
- lateral = head tilt

Superior rectus paresis results in a chin up posture.

Superior oblique paresis results in chin depression, turn towards and tilt away from the affected side.

Hess (Lees) screen and chart

The patient looks at a screen which has a grid marked on it, while the two eyes are dissociated (with red and green goggles and the use of red and green targets in the Hess, and by the use of two screens at 90° separated by a mirror which bisects their angle in the Lees). While one eye fixates a target in each of the positions of gaze, the projection of the target by the other eye is indicated by the subject. The position of this projection in each position of gaze is marked on a chart, which shows the position of each eye in the field of action of each muscle.

Paretic and restricted muscles are identified by their smaller excursion on the Hess chart, while the contralateral synergist has a correspondingly larger than normal excursion (secondary overaction).

The Hess chart is an important way of identifying a paretic muscle, and following the clinical course of the paresis. Surgical correction in paralytic and restrictive strabismus is undertaken when the Hess shows that the eye movements have become stable, or secondary contracture of the ipsilateral antagonist has begun.

Maddox rod

The Maddox rod is a complex lens comprising five adjacent cylinders of high power, usually of red glass. The effect of the adjacent cylinders is to create a streak image from a distant point light source perpendicular to the axes of the cylinders. This can be used to measure horizontal, vertical, and torsional deviations. Because the test is conducted using the trial frame, the angle of deviation can be measured readily by adding prisms to the trial frame to neutralize the separation between point and streak. Because the eyes are dissociated by the testing procedure, however, it cannot distinguish heterophoria from heterotropia.

Horizontal deviation

Place the Maddox rod in a trial frame before the right eye with cylinder axes horizontal: this eye will see a vertical red streak while the left will see the white point source. In orthophoria the streak will pass through the white point. In exodeviation the streak will be seen to the left of the point (crossed diplopia). In esodeviation the streak will be seen to the right of the point (uncrossed diplopia).

Measure the angle of deviation by placing sufficient prism before one eye (base-out for an esodeviation, base-in for an exodeviation) to cause the streak to pass through the middle of the point.

Vertical deviation

Place the Maddox rod in a trial frame before the right eye with cylinder axes vertical: this eye will see a horizontal red streak while the left will see the white point source.

In right hyperphoria the streak will be seen below the point. In left hyperphoria the streak will be seen above the point.

Measure the angle of deviation by placing sufficient prism before the right eye (base-down for right hyperphoria, base-up for left hyperphoria) to cause the streak to pass through the middle of the point.

Cyclodeviation

Place a red Maddox rod before the right eye and a white Maddox rod before the left. Rotate one until the subject reports that white and red streaks are superimposed in the same axis. The angular separation between the axes of the two rods is a measure of the cyclodeviation.

Sensory assessment of binocular function and diplopia

Simultaneous presentation of slightly disparate images to the two eyes produces a three-dimensional image if central mechanisms serving binocular fusion are intact. Retinal correspondence (normal = NRC, abnormal = ARC) refers to the relationship between the cortical projection value of corresponding points on each retina. ARC implies that the projection of points on one retina have become different from anatomically equivalent points on the other retina, as an adaption to avoid diplopia in strabismus. Stable binocular alignment depends on NRC and is absent in ARC. A stable result following squint surgery is therefore more likely if the patient has NRC.

Stereotests

Clinical stereotests are a quick and simple test of fusion capability. They indicate the minimal image disparity required for stereoscopic perception, and are an important determinant of the result of surgical correction of squint. The two eyes can be dissociated with coloured or polarizing filters, and presented with images of red and green, or opposite polarity (Wirt–Titmus, and TNO tests). Sensitivity to binocular disparity can be quantified by measuring ability to detect disparity between dots printed on either side of clear sheets of Perspex of various thicknesses (Frisby test).

Test of suppression

In the Worth four-dot test the eyes are dissociated by coloured goggles (red, right; green, left) while the subject looks at four illuminated coloured discs (two green, one red, one white). The white disc can be seen by either eye, but the red only by the right, and the green only by the left. The number of discs seen depends on binocular function:

- normal   four   (two green, one red, one red/green),
- R suppression   three   (all green),
- L suppression   two   (both red).

Test of abnormal retinal correspondence

Bagolini striped glasses are a pair of plano lenses with many parallel lines etched through the centre of each. These are placed before each eye in the trial frame with the etched lines perpendicular to each other (at 45° and 135°). They produce faint streaks through central fixation when a light is observed, without imposing artificial viewing conditions or dissociation.

The perception of the fixation light and streaks depends on binocular status and retinal correspondence:

- orthotropia, NRC   complete symmetric streak cross intersecting at the single light
- microtropia   as above, but with a gap in the centre of one streak (due to central suppression).
- esotropia > 10Δ, NRC   two uncrossed fixation lights, two uncrossed, complete streaks
- esotropia > 10Δ, ARC   one fixation light, symmetric streak cross (one streak fainter)
- exotropia   two crossed fixation lights, symmetric streak cross (central gap in one streak indicates ARC with suppression)

Test for postoperative diplopia

Surgical correction of longstanding strabismus, which may have become compensated by suppression or ARC, is sometimes followed by development or exacerbation of diplopia. Since this may be more troublesome than the original deviation, it is important to avoid surgery if postoperative diplopia is likely, and to warn patients of the possibility of postoperative diplopia before surgery. In the postoperative diplopia test, the effect of surgical correction is simulated by correcting the deviation measured objectively (by prism cover test) using prisms.

Postoperative diplopia is more likely in those with suppression in the presence of NRC of narrow fusional range. Although the patient with ARC may develop postoperative diplopia, cortical adjustment will compensate for the new eye positions, and diplopia will normally resolve—though in adults this may take several weeks.

Differential diagnosis of acquired ocular motility disorder

Clinical assessment of recently acquired extraocular muscle paresis should include investigation for hypertension and vascular disease, diabetes and dysthyroid disease, and demyelination and myasthenia, as appropriate. As well as assessment of ocular motility and binocular sensory function as described above, ocular examination should include optic disc inspection, and examination of the adjacent cranial nerves.

Referral for full neurological examination is indicated if the disorder is more extensive than an isolated vascular lesion involving one nerve, or if it progresses or fails to resolve. Pupil-involving III must be investigated immediately, since it may be caused by aneurysm or tumour, requiring neurosurgical management.

Causes of acquired ocular motility disorder

- neurogenic (ocular motor   vascular
  nerve lesion)   demyelinating
                              inflammatory
                              compressive

- myogenic   myasthenia gravis
                            ocular myopathy
- restriction   dysthyroid ophthalmopathy
                            trauma (blowout fracture)
                            inflammation (Brown's superior oblique tendon
                               sheath syndrome)
                            previous muscle surgery
                            previous retinal detachment surgery
- orbital   orbital mass restricting eye movement
- decompensated heterophoria (especially decompensation of exophoria
  following visual loss).

Neurogenic muscle paresis

Aetiology

1. III nerve paresis may be vascular (diabetes or hypertension), caused by aneurysm or tumour, or follow trauma or surgery. It presents with diplopia, exotropia, and ptosis. Pupil-involving (complete) III suggests aneurysm or tumour, and requires neurological assessment. External (pupil-sparing) III is usually vascular. Aberrant regeneration of III can lead to bizarre movements in the affected eye, sometimes including pupil anomalies.

2. IV nerve palsy commonly follows head injury, and is frequently bilateral. SO weakness causes diplopia either through the weakening of its depressing action (producing hypertropia), or through loss of intorsion. These effects are corrected surgically by recession of the ipsilateral IO, anteroplacement or tuck of the SO tendon at its insertion, or recession of the ipsilateral SR or contra-lateral IR, according to the clinical picture.

3. VI nerve palsy causes an incomitant esodeviation which may be reversible or irreversible. Vascular VI is common in arteriopaths; lateral rectus function generally recovers after 6–10 weeks. Diplopia is managed during recovery with Fresnel prisms stuck on to the spectacle lenses. Frequent reassessment permits the strength of the prisms gradually to be reduced as muscle function recovers.

Irreversible lateral rectus palsy may follow head injury, raised ICP, aneurysm, tumour, or neurosurgery. The patient adopts an abnormal head posture to reduce the diplopia. Some abduction (or at least, opposition of unopposed adduction) can be restored by Jensens's or Hummelsheim's procedure: MR is first weakened by recession or *Botulinum* toxin injection; in Jensens's procedure SR and IR are split longitudinally to provide strips of healthy muscle which are sutured to the similarly split paretic LR to augment its action, while its insertion is left in place; in Hummelsheim's procedure the lateral halves of SR and IR are mobilized and inserted into the superior and inferior margins, respectively, of the insertion of the paresed LR, which is itself left intact.

Dysthyroid ophthalmopathy

Dysthyroid ophthalmopathy is caused by an immunologically mediated chronic inflammatory infiltration of the muscles and other orbital structures. The diagnosis is confirmed by biochemical and serological tests and CT. Serology for antibody to thyroid microsomes is most commonly positive. There is muscle contraction in the early phase, later followed by contracture, restricting eye movements and producing incomitant strabismus. Inferior rectus is most commonly involved, producing elevation restriction, vertical diplopia, and an abnormal head posture with chin elevation. Other signs of dysthyroid ophthalmopathy (proptosis, corneal exposure, optic nerve compression) may coexist or be absent, and biochemical and immunological abnormalities, and goitre, are variable. Diplopia is corrected temporarily using Fresnel prisms on spectacles. The underlying endocrine dysfunction is referred for appropriate management. Muscle surgery may be undertaken to correct muscle imbalance when the Hess chart has been stable for 6–12 months.

Blowout fracture

Blunt trauma to the eye or orbit causing a blowout fracture (collapse of orbital floor or wall into an adjacent sinus) affects eye movements by causing prolapse of orbital tissues into the sinus. When an extraocular muscle or its associated fibrous sheath prolapses (usually inferior rectus or associated intermuscular septum into the maxillary antrum), or is trapped in the fracture, its action is weakened, and movement in the field of its antagonist is restricted. Clinical features of blowout include restriction of movement of the affected eye, usually in the vertical plane, surgical emphysema of the lids, and paraesthesia in the distribution of the infraorbital nerve; the diagnosis is confirmed by CT.

Early primary surgical reduction is indicated if the prolapse is large, causing marked enophthalmos, or if there is significant eye movement restriction. If soft tissue entrapment is less severe, the patient is managed conservatively, with serial Hess charts and prisms to correct diplopia, until the eye movements are stable enough to permit elective secondary corrective surgery.

Myasthenia gravis

Myasthenia is a disorder of neuromuscular conduction at the motor end plate. It can produce ocular motility disorder resembling any pattern of neurological lesion, including internuclear ophthalmoplegia, and should be suspected in all atypical or variable eye movement disorders. It may occur as an isolated ocular motor disorder (ocular myasthenia), or affect all striated muscle. Smooth muscle, and therefore pupil function, is not affected.

Myasthenia frequently occurs in conjunction with other autoimmune diseases, notably thyroid disease, and may be drug-induced, e.g. by penicillamine. Myasthenia secondary to malignancy (Eaton–Lambert syndrome) usually spares the extraocular muscles.

It commonly presents with ptosis or diplopia, which are variable, and increase in degree with fatigue. It is confirmed by the tensilon test, in which the eye movement response to tensilon (edrophonium, a short-acting anticholinesterase) is measured. Ptosis is measured, and/or extraocular movements plotted on the Hess chart. A test dose of 0.2 ml (2 mg) of tensilon is given intravenously through a cannula, and the patient is observed for 2 min for signs of excess parasympathetic stimulation. If there are no side-effects the remaining 0.8 ml are given, and the lids observed for temporary elevation, or the Hess chart repeated. Reduction in muscle weakness, which occurs within 1–5 min and may be short-lasting, confirms myasthenia. Atropine should be immediately available when tensilon is given, to counteract its muscarinic effects. Alternatively a trial of oral pyridostigmine may confirm the diagnosis, by giving symptomatic relief.

Progressive external ophthalmoplegia (PEO, ocular myopathy)

PEO is a disorder affecting the extraocular muscles but sparing the pupil, in which progressive symmetrical weakness of all extraocular movements occurs. Though initially the disorder is caused by muscle weakness, there is progressive contracture and fibrosis, producing restriction. Reflex movements (caloric stimulation, rotation, and Bell's phenomenon) are affected, distinguishing true PEO from pseudo-external ophthalmoplegia (caused by central supranuclear lesions, in which reflex movements are intact). PEO can occur in isolation (with or without levator and orbicularis weakness), or in conjunction with myopathic involvement of other muscles of the head and neck (usually inherited). It may be associated with pigmentary retinopathy, cardiac conduction defects and cerebral vacuolization (Kearns–Sayre syndrome, a non-familial mitochondrial disorder with onset during childhood).

Recommended further reading

Cashell, G.T.W. and Durran, I.M. (1981). *Handbook of orthoptic principles*, 4th edn. Churchill Livingstone, Edinburgh.

Diamond, G.R. and Eggers, H.M. (1993). *Strabismus and paediatric ophthalmology*. Vol. 5, *Textbook of ophthalmology* (ed. S.M. Podos and M. Yanoff.) Mosby, St Louis.

Mein, J. and Harcourt, B. (1986). *Diagnosis and management of ocular motility disorders*. Blackwell Scientific Publications, Oxford.

von Noorden, G.K. (1990). *Binocular vision and ocular motility*, 4th edn. Mosby, St Louis.

10
Paediatric ophthalmology

The same principles of ophthalmological history and examination apply to children as to adults, but there are important differences in emphasis. This is due partly to the different range of eye disorders presenting in children, and partly because clinical assessment of children's eyes, and measurement of their visual function, is limited by their understanding, tolerance, and cooperation.

History must often be obtained mainly from parents. Pay attention particularly to a parent's description of vision-dependent behaviour (responding, navigating, and manipulating), and always take a mother's concern about her infant's visual function seriously. The earliest signs of poor vision are behavioural, and may be subtle and indefinite. Babies less than a year old who never smile in response to mother's attention, and infants who do not make and hold eye contact, may fail to do so because their vision is very poor. The assessment of visual function in young children requires patience and careful observation. Orthoptists are skilled in measuring children's vision, and an orthoptic assessment, which includes tests of visual acuity, binocular vision, and eye movement, is an important part of the examination. Certain special investigations are especially useful in contributing to diagnosis when clinical assessment provides insufficient information. Electrodiagnosis is used to investigate retinal (electroretinography and electro-oculography) and retinostriate (visual evoked response) function. Ultrasound and CT scan examination are used to define the morphology and position of ocular, orbital, and intracranial pathology.

Assessment

History

Visual history

Visual behaviour
Parents of children with poor vision are usually aware of a problem, but may not always implicate the visual system. Their observation of an infant's behavioural capacity (reaching, manipulating, responding to facial expression, and smiling) is a very important clue to the possibility of visual pathology.

Squint
Parents often mean 'screwing up the eyes' when they speak of squinting. Establish what exactly is meant by squint, when it began, and whether it is intermittent or constant, unilateral or alternating.

Nystagmus
Roving eye movements in severe visual handicap are usually readily noticed by parents. The rapid conjugate horizontal movements of congenital nystagmus (CN), in which vision is less impaired, are sometimes noticed but thought to be normal.

Photophobia
Indicates lens or corneal opacity, ocular inflammation, buphthalmos, or cone disorder. It may be suggested by distress during examination, particularly indirect ophthalmoscopy.

Night blindness (nyctalopia)
Rod dysfunction, due to inherited (congenital stationary night blindness) disorder or vitamin A deficiency, causes nyctalopia. Vitamin A deficiency is rare in the West, but commonly accompanies malnutrition.

Both photophobia and nyctalopia may need to be asked for specifically (do they avoid bright lights and sunlight, or are they clumsy or disorientated in the dark?).

Birth history

Prematurity, mother's prenatal illness or medication, delivery (especially forceps delivery), and complications, may all be significant.

Family history

Ask whether there is any eye disorder in near relatives, especially siblings. Consanguinity increases the risk of recessively inherited disease. Myopia during childhood is a frequent cause of poor performance at routine school and pre-school acuity screening, and is often associated with myopia in one or both parents.

Inheritance

Inherited eye disorders frequently present during childhood.

Diseases with autosomal dominant inheritance have a 'vertical' presentation, in which 50 per cent of individuals in successive generations are affected.

Recessively inherited diseases are usually associated with more severe visual impairment, and the family history is 'horizontal'. In an affected generation, twenty-five per cent of individuals are affected and 50 per cent are carriers. Whole generations skip the condition completely, and it is unusual for a recessively inherited disease to affect successive generations. Consanguinity, especially if it is culturally widespread, increases the incidence of recessively inherited disease. Carriers are subclinically affected in some recessive and sex-linked disorders, and may show clinical signs of the disorder.

X-linked and mitochondrially inherited disorders affect males preferentially.

Penetrance and expressivity may be variable. Penetrance refers to the proportion of genotypically affected individuals who manifest a disease, and expressivity is a measure of the variability in the severity of a disease's clinical manifestation.

It is often useful to examine siblings and parents. Establishing the genetic background of a disease is not only diagnostically helpful, but also permits genetic counselling to be provided where appropriate.

General health

Congenital and genetic diseases affecting the eyes and vision sometimes have systemic manifestations. Consider general developmental progress and milestones, as well as possible CNS or metabolic disorder.

Examination

Ophthalmological examination of children should include an assessment of vision, eye movements and cover test, cycloplegic refraction and dilated fundus examination, together with such other examinations, tests, or investigations as individual cases may require.

Sensory examination

Vision and acuity

Uniocular visual loss is rarely symptomatic, but may present with strabismus.

Nystagmus indicates poor acuity, though it is not always present. As a guide, the coarser and slower and more 'roving' the nystagmus, the worse the visual function.

Babies

Most babies can hold steady fixation of a central target by 6 weeks or earlier, and follow a moving target at 2 months. Visually guided reaching occurs at 4 months, and by 6 months most babies can manipulate handled objects under visual control. By 1 year, visually guided behaviour includes scribbling and pointing.

Reflex tests of vision and ocular motility

Doubtful visual function can be tested by stimulating optokinetic nystagmus (OKN), and by observing the persistence or suppression of after-nystagmus following rotation (VOR). These reflex eye movements are stimulated through the pontine gaze centres, and have a visual input.

OKN is stimulated using an OKN drum, or a tape with vertical stripes or pictures. Intact OKN demonstrates function in the visual cortex, as well as intact supranuclear eye movement pathways. Lateralized cortical pathology causes defective OKN towards the side of the lesion. OKN appears to reverse in congenital nystagmus. Poor OKN response may have a motor as well as a sensory cause.

VOR is stimulated by rotating the infant held by the examiner. The normal VOR causes conjugate gaze deviation in the direction of rotation, can be suppressed if the child fixates the examiner, and ceases after only two or three beats when rotation stops. More sustained post-rotational after-nystagmus indicates poor cortical visual function.

Infants
Quantification of visual function in infants is difficult, but is particularly useful in assessing progressive improvement in those in whom vision is in question. Recognition, and visually guided reaching towards, small highly coloured attractive objects (100s and 1000s, smarties, etc.) gives a rough guide to visual function, but the acuity card procedure (ACP, a modified preferential looking test, to cards with spatial gratings of progressively higher frequency) is a more precise measure of acuity in infants too young to use other tests, and in mentally handicapped patients.

The Sheridan Gardner, K-pix, Landolt C, and illiterate E test are all modifications of Snellen testing, using standard types which do not require letter-naming. Most children over 3 years can manage the Sheridan Gardner test, and if there is doubt about a child's vision, observation should continue until a satisfactory Sheridan Gardner acuity has been obtained. Single letters presented at a distance of 6 m are matched by the child with those on a reference card. The Cambridge crowding cards are a modification in which the test letter is surrounded by others to assess amblyopia, in which acuity is reduced by visual crowding.

Visual fields

It is not possible to make formal visual field measurements in children, but patient observation of responses to toys and lights brought towards the centre from outside the visual field will generally indicate hemianopia.

Colour vision

Pseudo-isochromatic tests (Ishihara and others) are designed to investigate relative colour disorders affecting one or two of the three receptor types (red, green, and blue-sensitive). They are quick and easy to use, and are useful in screening for colour dysfunction.

The Farnsworth Munsell 100 hue test takes much longer, and requires considerably more attention from the subject. It is a more sensitive indicator of cone disorder, and reveals incomplete achromatopsia. The D15 is a restricted version of the same test, using 15 colours, which is more appropriate for children.

Binocular function

The images projected to the cortex by each of the two eyes are fused to produce stereoscopic vision. If this is present, it indicates that function is good in both eyes and in the cortex. Binocular function is poor if one eye is amblyopic or strabismic, and in the presence of cataract, posterior segment, optic nerve, or cortical pathology.

Tests of binocular function measure either its sensory or motor aspects. They are best observed and learned in the orthoptic department.

Sensory
Wirt–Titmus, TNO, Frisby, and other stereotests assess the cortical fusion of disparate images into a single perception of depth. Binocular disparity is achieved, respectively, by the use of polarization, red/green colour dissociation, or vertical separation of dots on either side of a perspex plate. The Wirt–Titmus fly test is a quick screening test, while TNO and Frisby measure stereoscopic function quantitatively, in seconds of arc.

Other tests of the sensory relationship between the two eyes include Bagolini striated glasses which are used to define central projection in free space, and the synoptophore, used to assess visual perception of separate images presented to each eye at controlled angles of deviation.

Motor
1. *20Δ prism test.* A 20Δ prism is placed base-out before one eye, while the eye is watched carefully for movement. The prism deviates the image to the temporal retina, and the eye must adduct in order to maintain binocular fixation. A brisk adducting movement indicates binocular function. If no adducting movement is made, the eye has poor (uniocular) vision or there is suppression, indicating poor binocular function.

2. *4Δ prism test.* Limited binocular function in the presence of a stable small angle squint (microtropia) is demonstrated by placing a 4Δ prism base-out before one eye, while observing carefully the movement of the other. The 4Δ prism deviates the image to a temporal parafoveal point. If there is good binocular function and no squint, the eye behind the prism makes a small adducting movement to refixate; the other eye first makes a conjugate abduction, followed by a compensatory refixating adducting flick. A microtropic eye has an area of suppression around central fixation, and because the 4Δ prism deviates the image into this 'suppression scotoma', no movement of either eye is made.

Ocular motility
The target used in ocular motility and cover testing must be small enough to represent a point in space, accommodative (i.e. not a simple point of light), and above all sufficiently interesting to command the child's attention. Testing should be performed with the target held at a distance of 0.3 m.

Eye movements

Test ductions and versions to the six cardinal positions, to elevation and depression, and to convergence. Watch particularly for:

1. Elevation in adduction (overacting inferior oblique).
2. Failure of elevation in adduction (Brown's superior oblique tendon sheath syndrome).

3. A and V patterns (change in the angle of deviation of a horizontal squint between elevation and depression).

4. Restriction, following muscle surgery.

5. Synkinetic movements: (a) lid movement of one eye on horizontal versions (Duane's lid-retraction syndrome); (b) lid elevation and depression on jaw movement (Marcus-Gunn jaw-winking syndrome).

6. Abnormal or bizarre movements of one eye (or its lids or pupil) on versions (aberrant III nerve).

7. Nystagmus.

Cover test

The cover test is a simple and powerful test of the muscle balance between the two eyes. If there is muscle imbalance, but it is compensated by good binocular function, the eyes remain straight as long as both are open (heterophoria, or latent squint). If compensation breaks down (in the absence of stable fusion), or is impossible (in the presence of muscle paresis) heterotropia (manifest squint), with diplopia or suppression, results.

Heterotropia (manifest squint) means that the visual axes of the eyes are not parallel when both are open.

Heterophoria (latent squint) means that the visual axes of the eyes are not parallel when they are dissociated, e.g. by occlusion.

Technique

The cover test requires an occluder and a fixation target. Purpose made occluders cover the eye with minimal distraction, and are better than a hand or a piece of paper. Cover testing is performed with and without spectacle correction, and at 0.3 and 6 m, to reveal any accommodative element.

1. *Stage 1: cover.* Cover one eye while watching the other. A refixation movement indicates that the unoccluded eye was not directed towards the target, taking up fixation when the fixing eye was covered. This is heterotropia (manifest squint). An abducting movement to refixate indicates *esotropia* (ET, convergent squint), whereas refixating adduction occurs in *exotropia* (divergent squint, XT).

2. *Stage 2: uncover.* Uncover an occluded eye, and watch for movement at the moment of uncover. Covering dissociates the eye (i.e. removes fusion of the two images). If the eyes had diverged on dissociation (latent divergent squint, *exophoria*, or XP) there will be an adducting movement on uncover as binocular vision is resumed. Similarly in EP (*esophoria*, latent convergent squint), the eye abducts on uncover. The uncover test may reveal less than the full angle of heterophoria.

3. *Stage 3: alternate cover.* Complete dissociation is achieved by alternate cover, revealing the full extent of heterophoria. The occluder is passed from one eye to the other every 0.5–1 s, at no time allowing simultaneous fixation by

both eyes. The movement of each eye is observed as it takes up fixation. The alternate cover test reveals the maximum angle due to combined latent and manifest squint.

4. The *prism cover test* (PCT) is a refinement of the alternate cover test, in which Perspex prism of graded strength on a bar are placed before one eye at uncover. The strength of the prism (in prism dioptres) which abolishes movement quantifies the full extent of the deviation.

Ocular examination

Red reflex

Inspect the reflex through each pupil using the retinoscope, or the direct ophthalmoscope (with its focusing wheel at zero). The normal reflex is clear red; in the presence of cataract, vitreous opacity, or posterior segment tumour it is dull or white.

Anterior segment

Most anterior segment abnormalities can be seen with good direct illumination angled obliquely. Use fluorescein to examine the cornea for ulceration. Slit-lamp examination is usually possible, with patience.

Gonioscopy (in buphthalmos) requires examination under anaesthetic.

Intraocular pressure

Applanation tonometry is not possible in most children except under anaesthetic. The handheld non-contact (Pulsair) tonometer can be used with children of any age.

Refraction

Cycloplegia (cyclopentolate 1 per cent, or 0.5 per cent under age 1, twice at 20 min intervals 20 min before refraction) is necessary under the age of 6 years or so. Atropine (oc. atropine 1 per cent daily for 3 days before refraction) is sometimes used, in children in whom cyclopentolate fails to produce satisfactory cycloplegia.

Subjective refraction is not usually practicable in children, and spectacles are ordered on the results of retinoscopy (making subtraction for the working distance, but not for cycloplegia).

Posterior segment

All children presenting with visual symptoms or squint should have a dilated fundus examination. Use the indirect ophthalmoscope, without excessive illumination, and a 28D lens to give a wide view including disc, macula, and post-equatorial retina. Greater magnification of areas of interest is given with the 20D, and the disc and macula can be examined with the direct ophthalmoscope.

Special investigations

Examination under anaesthesia

This is necessary if information of diagnostic importance cannot be gained while the child is awake. The opportunity should always be taken to carry out a refraction during EUA.

Indications

- Buphthalmos: gonioscopy, tonometry, corneal diameter, disc examination.
- Suspected retinoblastoma: complete bilateral fundus examination.
- Trauma: assessment, fundus examination, and exploration if necessary.

Electrodiagnostic tests

Electroretinogram (ERG)

The ERG derives from the neuroretinal response to light stimulus. The receptors drive the *a* wave, and the ganglion cells drive the *b* wave.

Recording is made from a gold leaf electrode in contact with the anaesthetized cornea over the lower lid, or a contact lens electrode. The stimulus is flash or flicker, in low (scotopic) and high (photopic) illumination, to stimulate, respectively, rods and cones.

Abnormalities of ERG response

- Extinguished ERG: Leber's amaurosis, Batten's disease.
- Increased amplitude *a* wave: albinism.
- Normal *a* wave, reduced *b* wave: congenital retinoschisis.
- Reduced photopic response, and response to flicker >20 Hz: achromatopsia.
- Reduced scotopic response: congenital stationary night blindness.

Electro-oculogram (EOG)

The EOG derives from retinal pigment epithelium (RPE) response to light stimulation.

Recording from electrodes at the medial and lateral canthi, the EOG records the potential difference between the back of the eye and the cornea in high and low illumination. The voltage measurement in the light divided by that in the dark (the light rise, or Arden index) is >185 per cent in normal eyes. It is reduced in the early stages of tapetoretinal degenerations, before the ERG is affected, and in Best's maculopathy.

Visual evoked response (VER)

The VER measures the velocity of conduction between the retina and cortex.

The latency (delay) between a flash or pattern stimulus, and the recording of its cortical response from scalp electrodes, is normally less than 120 ms. VER amplitude varies with recording conditions, and is a less useful measurement than latency. Cortical and visual pathway lesions cause abnormalities in VER, which are asymmetric in lateralized cortical disease. VER is also generally, but not invariably, reduced in diseases which reduce or abolish the ERG.

Radiology

CT scan provides high resolution views of structures which cannot be directly examined clinically; the posterior segment behind a cataract or other opacity, the orbit, and intracranial structures. Sedation or anaesthesia may be necessary. CT scans show anatomical structures and relations; diagnosis requires interpretation in the light of clinical information.

CT scan is particularly useful in investigating:

- Eye: tumour or mass; 75 per cent of retinoblastomas show radiological foci of calcification.
- Orbit: tumour (dermoid, haemangioma, lymphoma, rhabdomyosarcoma, neuroblastoma, medulloblastoma); inflammation (especially periosteal elevation over the ethmoid in orbital cellulitis); encephalocoele, meningocoele.
- Optic nerve: glioma, neurofibromatosis, optic nerve sheath meningioma.
- Intracranial: tumour, infarction, inflammation, ventricular dilatation, periventricular haemorrhage in low birthweight babies; exclusion of CSF obstruction before lumbar puncture.
- Trauma.

Ultrasound

B-mode ultrasonography gives a two-dimensional visualization of the eye and orbit, and is useful in assessing the integrity of posterior segment structures behind corneal or lens opacities, revealing a mass or retinal detachment. The main use of A-mode scan is used to measure the dimensions of ocular structures. It also provides a measure of sonic reflectivity and absorbance, which can help define tissue characteristics. Eyelid probes with gel-coupling are used.

Indications

Opacity or lid-swelling preventing inspection of the posterior segment.
Retrolental echoes are caused by:

- retinal detachment,
- vitreous haemorrhage,
- cyclitic membrane,
- choroidal detachment,
- retinoblastoma (irregularly echogenic due to focal calcification),
- granuloma,
- Coats' disease,
- persistent hyperplastic primary vitreous (PHPV).

Radiolucent intraocular foreign body.
Orbital examination, especially for tumour.

Refractive errors

The prescription of refractive correction in infants and children requires some judgement, and should not be undertaken simply because ametropia is found on refraction. It may be difficult to get an accurate refraction in an uncooperative child, even with cycloplegia, and an accurate assessment of visual acuity is often impossible. The prescription of an incorrect spectacle correction, or unnecessary glasses, should be avoided. Particular care should be taken in the prescription of corrections incorporating a high cylindrical component; unless the axis and power are precisely accurate the glasses may leave the child worse off, and it is often wise to undercorrect a cylinder.

1. *Hypermetropia.* In the presence of esotropia, prescribe the full cycloplegic correction In orthotropia, correct only if hypermetropia$> + 2D$. Consider bifocals for accommodative esotropes with high accommodative convergence/ accommodation ratio.

2. *Myopia.* Pre-school myopes generally need no correction unless $> - 1D$, or amblyopia. Correct school-age myopes, to help classwork.

3. *Astigmatism.* The effect of astigmatism on vision varies between individuals, and the tendency is for reduction in astigmatic error as the child grows. Errors $> 2D$ persisting beyond the age of 4 years, in the context of convincingly reduced acuity, should be corrected.

Concomitant strabismus (squint)

Deviation of the visual axis of one eye is common in children, and gives rise to functional (amblyopia) and cosmetic concerns. Concomitance refers to the constant angle of deviation measured in all positions of gaze, and contrasts with the incomitant deviation seen in paralytic strabismus, which is uncommon in children. Concomitant strabismus is usually associated with one or several of the following: accommodation, refractive error, poor binocular function, amblyopia; these are frequently interrelated (e.g. anisometropia may be associated with amblyopia, defective binocular function, and squint), and all must be considered in the course of management.

History

Age of onset influences functional prognosis. Early onset squints (before 18 months of age) are associated with poor binocular function, and the squinting eye may become densely and irreversibly amblyopic if not detected and treated early.

Intermittent squint may be of recent onset; in these cases binocular function is likely to be established, and only recently decompensated. Constant squint is more likely to be associated with amblyopia in the squinting eye.

Alternating squint implies equal, or nearly equal, visual acuity in each eye.

There is commonly a strong family history in children with squint, and 20–50 per cent of children with congenital or neonatal neurological disorder (cerebral palsy, hydrocephalus) have a squint.

Examination

Visual acuities

Measure using a technique appropriate to the child's age and capabilities.

Cover test

Identify the type of squint (eso- or exo-deviation, and the presence or absence of a vertical component) by cover test. The angle of deviation is measured by PCT. The deviation can also be seen by observation of the corneal reflexes of a bright hand-held light.

Eye movements

Look for muscle weakness or overaction.

1. Restriction of movement opposite the field of action of a muscle following surgery, and overaction of its contralateral antagonist, is due to fibrosis or excessive surgical resection.
2. Elevation of one or both eyes in adduction, common in esotropia, is due to inferior oblique overaction (or relative weakness of superior oblique).
3. Failure of elevation in adduction indicates superior oblique tendon trapping (Brown's syndrome).
4. Lid movements on versions occur in Duane's lid-retraction syndrome.
5. Lid movements on jaw movement, particularly lateral movements using the pterygoids, occur in the Marcus–Gunn jaw-winking syndrome.

Cycloplegic examination

Dilate the pupils with cyclopentolate 1 per cent × 2, for cycloplegic refraction and in order to examine the lenses and fundi (indirect ophthalmoscope). Posterior segment pathology (e.g. retinoblastoma, *Toxocara*, developmental optic nerve anomalies) can present with convergent squint.

Orthoptic examination and tests of binocular function

Orthoptists are skilled in the evaluation of many aspects children's visual function and ocular motility. Routine orthoptic examination of children includes cover test, PCT, examination of eye movements, motor and sensory assessment of binocular visual function, and the effect on the squint of accommodation and refractive correction. The ophthalmologist involved in the management of children with strabismus should be familiar with the theory and practice of tests of binocular function, which are best learned in the orthoptic department.

Clinical stereotests are a quick and simple test of fusion capability. They indicate the minimal image disparity required for fusion, and are an important determinant of the result of surgical correction of squint. The two eyes are dissociated, and presented with dissociated images (Wirt–Titmus and TNO tests). Sensitivity to binocular disparity can be quantified by measuring the ability of the eyes to detect disparity between dots printed on either side of sheets of Perspex of various thicknesses (Frisby test). Motor aspects of binocular fusion are quickly tested by the ability of one eye to overcome a 20Δ prism placed base-out before one eye, with both eyes viewing.

Classification of squint

Esodeviations

Esophoria (EP): latent convergent squint

Esotropia (ET)

Early onset (before 18 months)
Early onset ET is inevitably associated with defective binocular single vision, and commonly also with dissociated vertical deviation and latent nystagmus, and asymmetry of OKN.

Childhood (onset after 18 months)
- Convergence excess (near > distance deviation), caused by a high accommodative convergence:accommodation (AC:A) ratio.
- Fully accommodative (eliminated by full hypermetropic refractive correction).
- Partially accommodative.
- Non-accommodative.

Exodeviations

Exophoria (XP): latent divergent squint

Exotropia (XT)

1. *Intermittent XT.*
2. *Constant XT.*
3. *Convergence weakness*: deviation at near > distance.
4. *Basic XT*: deviation at near = distance.
5. *Divergence excess*: deviation at near < distance.
6. *Pseudo-divergence excess.* Resembles divergence excess, but shown to be truly basic XT on cover test following occlusion of the exotropic eye for 30 min, or with + 3.00DS lens: deviation at near = distance.
7. *Consecutive XT.* Complication of surgery to correct ET. Its onset may be delayed by years. Eyes with poor binocular function preoperatively, and amblyopic eyes, are especially likely to undergo secondary exodeviation.

A and V patterns

In A patterns, the eyes are more convergent in elevation than depression, often due to superior oblique overaction.

In V patterns, the eyes are more divergent in elevation than depression, usually due to inferior oblique overaction/superior oblique underaction (V eso), or superior rectus underaction (V exo).

Clinical symptoms occur most commonly in V ET and A XT.

Pseudo-squint

The following may resemble squint, but the cover test reveals no ocular deviation.

1. Broad epicanthic folds.
2. Negative angle kappa. The visual axis of the eye is displaced nasally (corneal reflexes displaced temporally) in pseudo-convergence. The reverse occurs in pseudo-divergence (positive angle kappa).
3. Telecanthus. Widely spaced medial canthi.
4. Hypotelorism. Narrow interpupillary distance.
5. Macular ectopia. Macula dragged horizontally by cicatrization following retinopathy of prematurity.

Management of squint

The aims of treatment are functional (to prevent or reduce amblyopia and to restore binocular visual function) and cosmetic (to achieve satisfactory stable ocular alignment). These aims are addressed in three stages:

1. Correction of refractive error.
2. Treatment of amblyopia.
3. Surgical correction.

Correction of refractive error

Hypermetropia

Without squint

Glasses are not generally ordered for hypermetropia < 2D before the age of 3–4 years. Intermittent squint is often eliminated with full hypermetropic correction. Above the age of 5 years, close work at school sometimes presents difficulty with an uncorrected hypermetropia > 2D.

With squint

The full correction is ordered (without an allowance for cyclopentolate cycloplegia). The commonest cause of incompletely corrected accommodative squint is incomplete refractive correction.

Myopia

Myopia should generally be fully corrected in children once they are at school. Undercorrection causes poor performance in distance acuity testing. Overcorrection may lead to accommodative esotropia.

Treatment of amblyopia

Occlusion of the better eye encourages the use of the amblyopic eye in tasks requiring visual attention. Occlusion is generally arranged daily for ½ days, and the resulting change in acuity monitored. Children with densely amblyopic eyes may resist occlusion, and its effectiveness depends to a large extent on the commitment of the parents. Occlusion is less effective in older children, and no reduction in amblyopia can be expected above 6–8 years old.

Successful occlusion improves acuity in the amblyopic eye. The squint alternates when the acuities of the two eyes are approximately equal, conferring a higher probability of surgical success.

Surgical correction

Surgery is indicated when squint persisting after refractive correction and treatment of amblyopia causes functional visual defect, or is cosmetically unsatisfactory.

Indications

Functional

The functional consequences of strabismus are amblyopia, and loss of (or failure to develop) binocular single vision. Surgical correction re-establishes the conditions for binocular single vision, and eliminates the cause of strabismic amblyopia.

The functional result of surgery to later-onset and intermittent squints is better than in constant or early-presenting squint, since binocular function has already developed, and amblyopia is more readily reversible.

Cosmetic

Constant large angle deviation is cosmetically unacceptable to children and parents. Surgery is indicated after refractive correction and occlusion therapy has reduced amblyopia in the squinting eye.

Timing of surgery

Early surgery is preferred in early-onset ET, in order to reduce the angle of deviation and reduce the inevitable amblyopia. The optimal timing of surgery is not clear. The greater surgical accuracy possible with older (and larger) eyes must be balanced against the greater amblyogenesis caused by delay, and surgery is usually undertaken between 1 and 2 years.

Surgery undertaken for functional indications is performed without delay, in order to minimize the loss of binocular single vision and the development of amblyopia. Maintenance of alignment following cosmetic squint surgery is most secure if it is visually reinforced, and it is ideal to operate when the squint alternates, i.e. when the acuity is equal in each eye.

Exodeviation

Exodeviation is less common than esodeviation in children. There is a spectrum ranging from XP (latent divergent squint) through intermittent XT to constant XT. Exodeviation may also be secondary to ocular disease, or consecutive, following previous surgery for convergent squint, though consecutive exodeviation usually appears after childhood. Convergence weakness in children is often treated satisfactorily by orthoptic exercises, but basic XT and divergence excess require surgery. There is less risk of amblyopia in divergent than in convergent squint.

The child with poor vision

Diagnosis depends on history, examination and assessment, and electrodiagnostics if necessary.

Severe visual impairment may be present at birth or acquired, and may be due to media opacity, or disorder of the retina or visual pathway (Table 10.1).

Educational implications, and possible genetic counselling, are important considerations in the management of children with visual handicap.

Congenital nystagmus (CN)

CN occurs as an isolated phenomenon, or in association with ocular or visual pathway disorder, except cortical blindness. Vision is usually impaired in the presence of nystagmus. The movements are slower and more wandering in severe visual failure, and faster, with smaller amplitude, in idiopathic CN with relatively good vision. Visual loss acquired after the age of 10 years is less likely to be associated with nystagmus. Oscillopsia does not occur in CN.

Latent nystagmus (LN) usually occurs in conjunction with infantile ET and dissociated vertical deviation; it occurs on unilateral occlusion, with its fast phase directed towards the fixing eye. Acuity with both eyes open is therefore considerably better than the acuity of either eye measured individually.

Assessment of CN

- record its pattern in different positions of gaze (see Chapter 8, p. 161),
- examine for iris transillumination (albinism),
- dilated fundus examination,
- cycloplegic refraction.

Electrodiagnosis may be necessary to investigate or exclude retinal disorder.

Table 10.1 Some causes of reduced vision in infants and children

	Vision	Presentation	Diagnosis
Congenital			
Persistent hyperplastic primary vitreous (PHPV)	poor	leucocoria, squint, cataract	pupil reflex, slit-lamp
Lens (cataract and ectopia) (lens opacities may also appear, or progress, after birth)	variable, uniocular or binocular	leucocoria, squint	slit-lamp, pupil reflex
Coloboma	variable, according to size and involvement of macula and optic nerve	reduced vision, squint	smooth-edged defect of variable size involving retina/choroid/iris/lens/lid
Leber's amaurosis	very poor	early (poor vision before age 1 year old) nystagmus, photophobia, sluggish pupils, late pigment retinopathy	absent ERG response
Achromatopsia	<6/24	nystagmus, photophobia, during infancy	ERG reduced photopic response; no response to flicker >20 Hz
Albinism	variable	photophobia	pale fundus; iris transillumination; high amplitude ERG a-wave
Optic nerve hypoplasia	poor if bilateral	poor vision if bilateral; squint at screening	disc (small, or 'double ring' sign); ERG normal; VER attenuated
Dominant optic atrophy	6/9–6/24	failed childhood vision tests	pale disc, especially temporal segment; affected relations
Cortical blindness	hemianopic or blind	low vision, often in babies with perinatal problems; no nystagmus	ERG normal; VER low amplitude, asymmetric or absent

	Vision	Clinical features	Investigations
Congenital nystagmus	6/9–6/60	nystagmus, abnormal head posture	VER delayed, ERG normal
Delayed visual maturation (DVM)	very poor initially spontaneous recovery at 4–8 months	blind baby, sometimes other CNS abnormalities, no nystagmus	
Acquired			
Corneal opacity	according to site, size, and density	trauma, ulcer (aphakia corrected by extended wear contact lens), viral and nutritional, buphthalmos inherited dystrophy	inspection
Lens (cataract and ectopia)	variable, uniocular or binocular	leucocoria, squint	slit-lamp, pupil reflex
Glaucoma (buphthalmos)	variable, decreasing as damage progresses	large eye, photophobia, lacrimation	inspection, examination under anaesthesia, gonioscopy, tonometry
Juvenile Batten's disease	progressively poor	acquired visual loss age 5–6 years, mental changes, nyctalopia	VER low amplitude or absent, ERG low b wave, EEG abnormal, vacuolated lymphocytes
Posterior segment inflammation	variable	poor vision, squint	ophthalmoscope
Hydrocephalus	variable	monitoring hydrocephalus	
Optic neuritis	acutely reduced, usually uniocular	usually febrile illness	delayed VER
Optic nerve compression	variable	squint	disc swelling, CT ophthalmoscope
Macular dystrophy	variable	reduced vision	
Meningitis, encephalitis	variable	reduced vision during illness	

Causes of CN

- idiopathic (unassociated)
- with ocular disorder   congenital cataract
  albinism
  achromatopsia
  Leber's amaurosis, retinitis pigmentosa and its variants
  optic nerve hypoplasia
  optic nerve glioma.

Nystagmus due to CNS disorder (vestibular and central nystagmus) sometimes occurs in children. There are usually other neurological signs.

Watering eyes

Watering eyes are common during the first year of life, causing intermittent or constant sticky discharge, which becomes recurrently infected. The tearing may be due to outflow obstruction, or secondary to ocular surface disorder.

Secondary tearing may be caused by irritation due to a corneal or subtarsal foreign body, inflammation or infection, or contact lens. Lacrimation, together with photophobia, is a common presenting symptom of buphthalmos.

The lacrimal drainage system usually becomes patent before birth. Functional patency of either the canaliculi or the nasolacrimal duct may be delayed, however, causing epiphora and accumulation of lacrimal secretions. Probing and syringing (usually through the upper canaliculi) should be arranged if the problem has not resolved spontaneously (as it often does) by 9 months or so.

Cataract

Aetiology

- inherited
  cataract alone (dominant, recessive, sex-linked)
  chromosome abnormalities (Down's and Turner's syndromes)
- with inherited metabolic disorder hypocalcaemia
  galactokinase deficiency (well infants)
  galactosaemia (sick infants)
  hyperglycaemia
  hypoglycaemia
  Lowe's syndrome
- maternal infection
  rubella
  varicella
  cytomegalovirus
  Toxoplasma

- inflammatory   uveitis (e.g. in juvenile rheumatoid arthritis)
- developmental ocular anomalies anterior polar cataract
             aniridia, cleavage syndromes
             retinitis pigmentosa
             PHPV
             ROP
- drug induced   steroids
- trauma
- idiopathic

Management

The management of cataract in infancy and childhood includes investigation of aetiology, assessment of the visual effect of the cataract, and the decision whether to operate. When surgery is indicated consideration must be given to the appropriate surgical technique, the optical management of aphakia, and minimization of amblyopia. It is particularly difficult to avoid amblyopia in uniocular cataract, and because the visual results following surgery of uniocular cataract are usually poor, surgical intervention is often confined to infants with bilateral cataracts.

Assessment

Aetiology
The commonest aetiological associations of infantile cataract are listed on p. 271.

Since progression of lens opacification can be arrested in some (e.g. galacto-kinase deficiency), and treatment of the underlying condition is important in others, it is important to exclude or confirm these disorders in an infant with cataract.

Visual function and the decision to operate
It is very difficult objectively to measure visual function in young infants. The decision to operate depends on an assessment that vision will be better following surgery, with its attendant risks, and the difficulties of optical correction and amblyopia therapy, than it would have been without surgery. This decision is based on the morphology and density of the cataract, the visual behaviour of the patient, and the performance in tests of vision, such as preferential looking.

Surgery

Once the decision to operate has been made, surgery is undertaken without delay. Vitrectomy-instrumented lensectomy is the procedure of choice below the age of 2 years, since postoperative capsule opacification is vigorous in these eyes, and also in the presence of PHPV. Aspiration may be undertaken in older eyes. The second cataract should be removed within a week of the first, the first being occluded in the interim, in order to minimize amblyogenesis. Give topical steroid and atropine postoperatively to prevent synaechia formation.

Optical correction and amblyopia

Immediate and frequently repeated refraction, correction with gas permeable contact lenses up to the age of 2–3 years, or glasses thereafter, and occlusion therapy, are essential to prevent amblyopia. Soft contact lenses are fitted simultaneously at the conclusion of surgery to the second eye following bilateral congenital cataract extraction; they are usually overcorrected by 3D to focus the near world.

Intraocular lens implants in children are controversial, and they are not widely used.

Ectopia lentis (dislocated lens)

Signs

- iridodonesis,
- visible lens edge,
- rapid change in refraction, especially changing cylinder.

Aetiology

- congenital ectopia lentis (autosomal dominant),
- Marfan's syndrome,
- homocystinuria,
- Weill–Marchesani syndrome,
- spherophakia,
- trauma.

Management

Conservative

A lens fully dislocated into the vitreous is well tolerated, but may cause uveitis or glaucoma. Anterior dislocation may cause pupil block, producing high pressure, pain, and corneal oedema. An isolated episode is treated with mydriatics; recurrent pupil block caused by a mobile ectopic lens requires definitive treatment by lensectomy.

Surgical

Indications
- reduced acuity (lens edge in visual axis),
- cataract,
- lens-induced uveitis,
- pupil block,
- glaucoma,
- retinal detachment.

Complications
- retinal detachment,
- general anaesthesia hazard in homocystinuria.

Retinal disorders in children

Inherited retinal disorders are not common, but they generally present in childhood, and must therefore be considered in a child with poor vision or nystagmus.

Albinism

Albinism may affect the eyes alone (ocular albinism, X-linked), or the eyes and skin (oculocutaneous albinism). Oculocutaneous albinism is further classified into tyrosinase positive and tyrosinase negative subgroups, according to *in vitro* tyrosinase activity in incubated hair root bulbs.

Clinical features
- reduced vision,
- nystagmus,
- photophobia,
- iris transillumination,
- foveal aplasia,
- pale fundus,
- ERG high amplitude *a* wave.

Vision is most profoundly affected in tyrosinase negative albinism, in which hair and skin are completely unpigmented. Tyrosinase positive albinos are less severely affected, retaining variable skin and hair pigmentation. They may present with nystagmus.

Achromatopsia

- congenital defective or absent cone function
- clinical presentation   reduced visual acuity (6/36–3/60)
  photophobia
  nystagmus
  refractive error (usually hypermetropic)
  profound panspectral colour defect
  normal fundus in infants and young children
  later a bull's-eye-like maculopathy develops
- ERG   absent response to flicker >20 Hz
  reduced or absent photopic ERG
- treatment   refractive correction, with strong tint to relieve photophobia

X-linked congenital retinoschisis

The macular retina is split between receptors and ganglion cells, and there is peripheral schisis in 50 per cent. There is an abnormal sheen in the deep vitreous, or at the vitroretinal interface. Visual impairment is variable, and may be progressive. Occasionally the schisis ruptures a retinal blood vessel, causing vitreous haemorrhage. Electrodiagnostic tests show an enlarged ERG a wave, with attenuation of the b wave.

Retinitis pigmentosa and other tapetoretinal degenerations

These are inherited retinopathies in which progressive degeneration of both neurosensory retina and RPE causes progressive visual loss. Inheritance may be dominant, recessive, or sex-linked; vision is affected least in dominant and most in recessive forms.

Onset of symptoms in retinitis pigmentosa usually occurs during late childhood. Variants occurring in younger children include Leber's amaurosis (vision severely affected at birth or shortly afterwards), Usher's syndrome (associated with deafness), Refsum's syndrome, and congenital stationary night blindness.

Electrodiagnostic tests are particularly helpful in studying tapetoretinal degenerations. The EOG light rise (Arden index) is always reduced early, usually before the onset of clinical abnormalities. The ERG a wave becomes attenuated in all, but in Leber's amaurosis the entire ERG response is grossly attenuated or flat from birth.

Neurolipidoses

Unusual disorders of lipid storage affecting retina and CNS, and sometimes cornea.

Juvenile Batten's disease is an uncommon autosomal recessive disorder presenting with poor vision during childhood; bull's-eye maculopathy, fits and progressive dementia follow. Diagnosis is made by electron microscopic finding of 'fingerprint-like' inclusions in neurones obtained at rectal biopsy, and lymphocytes, which are vacuolated.

Other neurolipidoses include Tay–Sachs disease, sialidosis, and Niemann–Pick disease, which present with poor vision, dementia and epilepsy, and a cherry red spot at the macula.

Retinopathy of prematurity (ROP)

Premature birth confers risk of peripheral retinal fibrovascular proliferation, which may lead to visual impairment or (now rarely) blindness. The precise relationship between oxygen therapy and ROP is not clear; vessel narrowing may accompany oxygen therapy, followed by ischaemia and proliferation when the oxygen partial pressure is subsequently reduced. Low birthweight premature infants, and those whose neonatal course is complicated by infection or haemorrhage, are at increased risk.

Examine for ROP through dilated pupils, using the indirect ophthalmoscope with a 28D lens, and a paediatric lid speculum and scleral depressor.

Clinical staging of ROP

Stage 1: Demarcation line at anterior limit of normally vascularized retina.
Stage 2: Ridge at anterior limit of normally vascularized retina.
Stage 3: Extraretinal neovascularization on ridge.
Plus disease: Stage 3 plus engorgement of retinal or iris vessels, vitreous haze.

The threshold (for treatment) is reached when there are 5 or more contiguous or 8 or more cumulative clock hours at stage 3 in the post-equatorial retina, in the presence of plus signs. Treatment of these eyes with cryotherapy reduces the risk of epiretinal membrane formation, and progression to cicatrizing disease by 50 per cent. Photocoagulation, using the indirect ophthalmoscope laser, is increasingly used as an alternative to cryotherapy.

Complications of ROP

- myopia,
- dragged disc and macular ectopia,
- tractional retinal detachment.

Infections

Toxoplasma

Toxoplasma gondii is a protozoan parasite whose definitive host is the cat. Infection may be congenital or acquired, and is frequently subclinical. Ocular toxoplasmosis presents with foci of retinochoroiditis, which are irregular flat yellowish fundus lesions, with pigment clumping and overlying vitritis. Recurrent lesions occur around scars as 'satellites'.

Toxocara

Toxocara canis is an acquired nematode infestation contracted by ingesting dirt contaminated by infected puppy faeces. If the migrating larval worm reaches the eye, a focal inflammation results, causing granular uveitis, and serious visual impairment.

Clinical features:

- leucocoria,
- uveitis,
- visual loss,
- squint,
- elevated granuloma (usually at the posterior pole).

Diagnosis is confirmed by serology.

Orbital disease

Inflammation

Inflammation involving orbital tissues is divided into preseptal and postseptal compartments by the orbital septum, a thin fibrous sheet joining the tarsal margin with the orbital rim.

Orbital (postseptal) cellulitis

Aetiology

Sinus infection (usually ethmoid sinus in children, due to *Haemophilus influenzae*).

Clinical features

- pain and proptosis,
- restricted eye movements,
- conjunctivitis and periocular inflammation,
- reduced vision,
- fever.

Management

- CT scan: look for sinus disease, periosteal elevation, orbital abscess.
- Swab conjunctiva and nasopharynx.
- ENT surgical opinion; surgical drainage of infected sinus may be necessary.
- Treat with intravenous antibiotics, including agents active against staphylococcus, Gram negative, and anaerobes (e.g. chloramphenicol or gentamicin and cefuroxime, and metronidazole).

Complications

Posterior extension causing cavernous sinus thrombosis, meningitis, and cerebral abscess.

Preseptal cellulitis

Aetiology

Rapidly increasing superficial infection of lids or adjacent skin. Commonly begins as an insect bite or sting, or stye.

Clinical features

- Swelling, which may be considerable, making examination of the eye difficult.
- No proptosis.
- Eye movements normal.

Management

- swab,
- oral broad spectrum antibiotic.

Complications

Abscess.

Orbital tumour

Orbital tumours cause proptosis and ocular displacement. Relative afferent pupil defect indicates optic nerve compression or invasion, and restriction of eye movements may be caused by restriction, muscle infiltration, or motor nerve involvement. Dilated fundus examination may show optic nerve head swelling or atrophy, or choroidal folds.

Presentation

- proptosis (axial proptosis suggests intraconal mass),
- squint,
- diplopia,
- extraocular movement restriction,
- reduced vision.

Differential diagnosis

- encephalocoele,
- dermoid,
- capillary haemangioma,
- optic nerve glioma,
- optic nerve sheath meningioma,
- teratoma,
- rhabdomyosarcoma,
- Hodgkin's disease and leukaemia,
- neuroblastoma.

Benign tumours cause slowly progressive proptosis, opticociliary shunt vessels at the disc, and radiological enlargement of the orbit, whereas malignant tumours cause rapid progression and erosion of the orbital walls.

Glaucoma

Glaucoma with onset during infancy is called buphthalmos, and is usually caused by congenital angle anomaly. The sclera and cornea are more elastic in infants than in older eyes, and reduced drainage facility at this age causes distension of the eye as well as optic nerve head damage. The horizontal corneal diameter (HCD) provides an objective measure of progressive enlargement, and the response to treatment, at an age when accurate visual field measurement is not possible.

Buphthalmos is bilateral in 65 per cent, but usually asymmetric. Anterior chamber cleavage anomalies represent imperfect separation of the embryonic mesoderm which forms corneal stroma, anterior iris and trabecular meshwork, and result in a drainage angle which is malformed or covered in primitive mesoderm. Inheritance is recessive in 20 per cent and sporadic in 80 per cent.

Buphthalmos often presents initially with lacrimation and photophobia. It is important to exclude buphthalmos in children presenting with these symptoms, and not to assume that they are caused by conjunctivitis or blepharitis.

Aetiology

Anterior chamber cleavage syndromes (posterior embryotoxon, Axenfeld's anomaly, Peter's anomaly, Rieger's syndrome, and aniridia) represent a spectrum of patterns of anomaly involving drainage angle, corneal endothelium, iris and anterior lens surface. Glaucoma is a characteristic feature of all. It may also occur in Sturge–Weber syndrome (congenital haemangiomas, in the trigeminal distribution and intracranially), neurofibromatosis, and in the presence of an intraocular tumour.

Clinical features

- photophobia,
- lacrimation,
- redness,
- enlarged cornea (HCD > 10.5 mm),
- cloudy cornea (decompensation),
- breaks in Descemet's membrane (Haab's striae).

Differential diagnosis

Large cornea

- uniocular myopia,
- megalocornea,
- keratoglobus,
- contralateral nanophthalmos.

Cloudy cornea

- corneal dystrophy,
- mucopolysaccharidosis,
- interstitial keratitis.

Corneal striae

Birth injury.

Management

Gonioscopy, HCD, and IOP measurement are carried out under anaesthetic. Surgical division of mesoderm occluding the angle (goniotomy), is performed at the same time; trabeculotomy, trabeculectomy or tube and plate drainage are occasionally performed. Examination under anaesthesia is repeated at intervals, to ensure that HCD and IOP are stable.

Retinoblastoma

Retinoblastoma is the commonest malignant intraocular tumour in children. It usually presents within the first 3 years, and never above 6 years old.

Inheritance is autosomal dominant with incomplete penetrance, or sporadic. The risk that unaffected parents without a family history will produce a second affected child is 6 per cent, and the risk of a third affected child is 50 per cent. Bilateral retinoblastoma always has an inherited basis. Knudson's two-hit theory proposes that retinoblastoma follows a succession of two genetic insults. In inherited cases the first 'hit' is present in germinal DNA, so that all primitive retinal cells are defective; a second hit may involve more than one cell, and tumours are therefore commonly multiple and occur early. In sporadic disease both hits involve the DNA of a somatic (primitive retinal) cell; sporadic retinoblastoma therefore does not present as young as inherited disease, and the offspring of survivors are not at high risk. Twenty per cent of patients with retinoblastoma develop another malignancy in early adult life.

Presentation

- leucocoria
- poor vision
- squint
- 'anterior uveitis' masquerade   red eye
                                    pseudohypopyon (tumour cells)
- secondary glaucoma and corneal oedema
- signs caused by extraocular and secondary spread

Clinical features

Dilated examination of *both* eyes under anaesthetic shows a single or multifocal white fundus mass. This may be confined to the retina, or extend into the vitreous (endophytic), with surface blood vessels and 'seedling' cells in the vitreous. Intralesional calcification is typical and is seen well on CT scan.

Treatment

Retinoblastoma is uncommon, and is best managed in units with specialist experience. Enucleation of the affected eye, or of the more severely involved eye together with radiotherapy to the other eye, is combined with chemotherapy. Three-year survival of the presenting tumour in specialist units can be as high as 90 per cent.

Recommended further reading

Harley, R.D. (1983). *Paediatric ophthalmology*, 2nd edn. W.B. Saunders, Philadelphia.

Isenberg, S.J. (1989). *The eye in infancy*. Year Book Medical Publishers, Chicago.

Krill, A.E. (1972). *Hereditary retinol and choroidal diseases*, Vol. 1. Harper & Row, Hagerstown.

Krill, A.E. and Archer, D. (1977). *Krill's hereditary retinal and choroidal diseases*, Vol. 2. Harper & Row, Hagerstown.

Taylor, D. (1990). *Paediatric ophthalmology*. Blackwell, Oxford.

Wybar, K. and Taylor, D. (1983) *Paediatric ophthalmology*. Marcel Dekker, New York.

11
Ocular trauma

Assessment

Assessment of the extent of tissue damage following injury to or around the eye requires a detailed history and a full systematic examination. Serious injuries are not necessarily accompanied immediately by visual symptoms. The consequences of missing perforation or retained intraocular foreign body (IOFB) can be disastrous, and can only be avoided by suspecting and excluding these complications whenever they are a possibility.

History
Record precisely how and in what circumstances the injury was sustained, the nature of any materials involved, and any preceding eye or visual history.

Examination
Test visual acuity and pupil reactions; carry out external inspection, slit-lamp and ophthalmoscopic examination, and assess the extraocular movements. Sketch the site and extent of injuries, and photograph them if appropriate.

If periorbital oedema makes anterior segment examination difficult, separate the lids gently with a Desmarre's retractor under topical anaesthetic. Examination under anaesthetic and exploration may be necessary if the full extent of the injury still cannot be assessed.

Investigation
Assess for bony orbital injury and suspected IOFB by X-ray or CT scan. Ultrasound demonstrates lens disruption and retinal detachment obscured by haemorrhage, and reveals an IOFB by its high sonic reflectivity.

X-ray must always be taken for IOFB following high risk injury (hammering, especially on to metal, and accidents involving high-speed machinery).

Classification of ocular trauma

Superficial
The eyelids give protection from low velocity injuries, and are involved in chemical and thermal burns. Injury to the ocular surface causes pain, blepharospasm and photophobia, reflex pupil spasm, and secondary anterior uveitis.

Closed
Blunt injury to the eye or face may cause a blowout fracture of the orbital floor,

Le Fort facial fracture, rupture of the globe, lens dislocation, angle recession, intraocular haemorrhage, retinal oedema, or retinal dialysis.

Penetrating

Penetrating injury carries a high risk of sight-threatening complication due to:

- infection,
- intraocular tissue disruption,
- uveitis,
- haemorrhage,
- phthisis.

Retained IOFB causes chronic inflammation, scarring, and traction; those containing iron or copper also cause direct chemical toxicity. IOFB should be suspected, and confirmed or excluded radiographically, in any injury following high velocity impact.

Superficial trauma

Damage to the eyeball must be excluded in all cases of lid injury. Exposure keratopathy is a risk when lid closure has been compromised.

Lid laceration

Assess whether the laceration has involved the full thickness of the lid, the lid margin, the puncta or canaliculi. Exclude perforation of the eyeball, exploring conjunctival lacerations before closing them. Using topical and infiltrated (lignocaine 2 per cent + adrenalin) anaesthetic, clean and debride the wound thoroughly to expose its full extent and remove any clot or foreign matter. Suture in layers, using 6.0 absorbable suture to conjunctiva, tarsal plate and orbicularis, and 6.0 prolene to appose lid margins perfectly, and to skin.

Canalicular division is best repaired as a primary procedure under the operating microscope; the canalicular ends are sutured around a silastic (e.g. Crawford tube) passed through the punctum to bridge the break. Identification of the medial end of the divided lower canaliculus by probing the intact upper canaliculus with a pigtail probe may lead to stenosis, further compromising drainage, and should be avoided if possible.

Lid injuries with severe tissue loss which will require reconstructive surgery are best cleaned and stabilized in the first place, so that definitive repair can be performed when surgical conditions are optimal. Corneal exposure is prevented by temporary occlusion of defects with ointment and paraffin gauze.

Burns

Thermal and chemical burns cause similar patterns of tissue injury; thermal damage, however, is immediate, while the effects of chemical burns may be prolonged.

Chemical burns

Pathology

Acids coagulate protein, limiting the depth of tissue injury they cause. Caustic alkalis form lipid soluble soaps which facilitate deeper penetration, and therefore cause deeper, prolonged, and progressive damage. Alkali burns are characterized by conjunctival blanching due to acute ischaemia, anterior uveitis, and raised intraocular pressure (IOP).

Immediate management

Chemical burns must be copiously and continuously irrigated until no chemical agent remains. Litmus testing (using multitest analysis sticks) can be used to indicate residual acid or alkali. Treat acute caustic alkali burns with topical antibiotic, steroid (hourly in severe cases), and atropine, and oral ascorbate. If the corneal epithelium has been lost, a bandage contact lens should be fitted; corneal graft may be necessary if perforation is imminent, or as a secondary elective procedure when corneal re-epithelialization is complete. Grafts in these eyes are at high risk of failure due to rejection. Skin grafting may be necessary following extensive burns to prevent cicatrizing scars.

Delayed complications

Loss of conjunctival goblet cells, and cicatrization, may develop as delayed complications of burns involving the conjunctiva, especially chemical burns. Tear film instability and entropion contribute to exposure keratopathy and progressive corneal scarring.

Ultraviolet burns

Superficial burns may be caused by unprotected exposure to sun-lamps or welding flash ('arc eye'), and prolonged exposure to sunshine reflected by snow. Topical anaesthesia may be necessary to relieve blepharospasm and allow examination of the anterior segment.

Symptoms

- pain,
- photophobia,
- reduced vision.

Signs

- lid erythema and swelling,
- ciliary injection,
- corneal superficial punctate keratopathy, oedema, epithelial ulcer,
- anterior uveitis.

Treatment

- cycloplegia,
- antibiotic ointment,
- topical steroid if there is corneal oedema and anterior uveitis.

Conjunctiva

Foreign body

Superficial foreign bodies frequently lodge beneath the upper tarsal plate or in the lower fornix; if loose they are washed by tear currents to the medial canthus. Evert the upper lid and inspect the fornices, and remove a foreign body using a cotton wool bud or needle at the slit-lamp, or by irrigation.

Laceration

Conjunctiva may be lacerated following either sharp or blunt trauma. Following fragmentation injuries (e.g. broken glass) inspect the inferior fornix and clear it of retained foreign bodies. Exclude perforation of the globe beneath a conjunctival laceration; if necessary arrange to explore the wound surgically.

Repair uncomplicated conjunctival laceration under local anaesthesia using absorbable suture (6.0 gut or 8.0 vicryl).

Cornea

Corneal abrasion

Fluorescein staining demonstrates the extent and depth of an abrasion. Re-epithelialization is usually complete in 2 days. Treat with antibiotic ointment and cycloplegia.

Corneal erosion

Corneal erosion is a common recurrent sequel to epithelial trauma, which presents with foreign body sensation, blepharospasm, and photophobia, often on waking.

Treat symptomatically with ointment, and if necessary cycloplegia and a pad for a day or two, while the erosion re-epithelializes.

Corneal foreign body

Metallic corneal foreign bodies commonly follow metal grinding. Most can be lifted from the surface of the anaesthetized cornea with a sterile needle at the slit-lamp. The residual rust ring is easier to remove after a few days, when it is less friable.

If a corneal foreign body has penetrated deeply into the stroma, exclude perforation by Siedel test.

Closed trauma

Closed trauma follows blunt injury to the eye or face. Exclude rupture of the globe by clinical examination, and if necessary by CT scan and exploration. Rupture following blunt injury usually occurs around the rectus muscle insertions or at the limbus, but as the orbital floor is generally the weaker structure, orbital blowout fracture is commoner than scleral rupture.

Anterior segment

Hyphaema

Blunt trauma commonly causes intraocular haemorrhage from ruptured iris vessels; blood collects in the anterior chamber and settles to form a hyphaema. Red cells can be distinguished from inflammatory cells by their smaller size and lesser reflectivity. Uncomplicated hyphaema settles with rest; in-patient treatment is probably not necessary if the hyphaema is small, the IOP is not elevated, and adequate rest at home can be assured. There is some evidence that treatment with topical steroids may reduce the risk of secondary haemorrhage.

Sphincter rupture (causing traumatic mydriasis) iridodialysis, and angle recession are complications of blunt trauma, and may accompany hyphaema. They generally cause no symptoms, but angle damage may lead to glaucoma.

Secondary haemorrhage occasionally occurs as a delayed (2–6 days following the initial injury) complication, filling the anterior chamber with blood, and causing pupil block glaucoma. Haemoglobin is reduced in the ischaemic environment caused by the raised pressure, giving the anterior segment a uniformly dark or black appearance. Failure to reduce the pressure and clear the anterior chamber of clot leads to irreversible staining of the posterior cornea by haemoglobin. Treat secondary haemorrhage using intensive mydriatic to relieve the pupil block, together with topical steroid, and intravenous acetazolamide to reduce the IOP. Surgery (peripheral iridectomy and aspiration of the clot) may be necessary.

Lens

Lens opacification may follow ocular trauma of any kind. It varies in degree from inconsequential to dense cataract, and may be immediate, or delayed by years.

Lens-associated uveitis (phacotoxic and phacoanaphylactic) has an increased incidence in eyes with traumatic cataract; treat acutely with steroids and mydriatics, and definitively by extracapsular cataract extraction.

Subluxation and dislocation

Zonule rupture causes subluxation or dislocation of the lens, either anteriorly or posteriorly. Visual acuity is impaired in either case by the optical effect of ectopia; in addition anterior dislocation causes pupil block, while posterior dislocation into the vitreous may cause uveitis or glaucoma.

Treat pupil block by intensive mydriasis. If this is unsuccessful, or the problem becomes recurrent, surgical lensectomy, sometimes combined with trabeculectomy, may be necessary. If the lens has subluxed there may be disruption of the drainage angle, seen by gonioscopy. Medical treatment, using steroid and mydriatic, may be sufficient to manage an eye with a posteriorly dislocated lens. If uveitis or glaucoma is unmanageable medically, the lens may need to be removed; in this case a vitrectomy procedure will be necessary.

Posterior segment

Traumatic retinal dialysis

Disinsertion of the retina at the ora serrata due to trauma is caused by momentary deformation of the eye during an antero-posterior compression injury (e.g. a blow by a ball or a fist). Both tangential and perpendicular forces are exerted on the vitreous base, which is firmly attached to the pre-equatorial retina; a segment of this may then be torn from the ora serrata and elevated into the vitreous as a 'bucket-handle'. The presence of such a peripheral bucket-handle distinguishes a traumatic dialysis from the commoner idiopathic dialysis, and from a giant tear. The break left by the retinal tear should be closed by external buckling to prevent or repair retinal detachment.

Vitreous haemorrhage (VH)

VH following closed trauma is likely to be associated with a retinal tear. Exclude or confirm retinal detachment (Table 11.1). If there is no retinal detachment, manage by observation while the haemorrhage clears, and consider vitrectomy

Table 11.1 Signs of retinal detachment in the presence of vitreous haemorrhage

Relative afferent pupil defect
VH without retinal detachment does not cause RAPD
Projection of light
Projection is accurate to four quadrants if retina is attached, but inaccurate if it is detached. Only very dense VH compromises projection in the absence of retinal detachment
Indirect ophthalmoscope examination
Ultrasound scan (B-mode)
Carry out B-scan, watching the movement of the posterior echogenic face, to distinguish retinal from posterior hyaloid echo. Retinal detachment gives a mobile echogenic face which is inserted at the optic disc (unlike the echo given by the posterior hyaloid face, which is not attached at the disc, but peripherally at the vitreous base). Having the patient move the eyes up and down or side to side (dynamic scan) often helps distinguish retinal from vitreal echoes

if the vitreous fails to clear in 2 months. VH in the presence of retinal detachment requires early surgery to close breaks and reattach the retina.

Commotio retinae

Rapid vessel compression and decompression following trauma cause capillary rupture and increased permeability, leading to preretinal, nerve fibre layer, and intraretinal haemorrhage, and oedema. Involved retina appears pale and thickened.

Commotio resolves over a period of weeks without treatment, but macular involvement causes reduced visual acuity which may persist, sometimes in the presence of a macular hole.

Choroidal rupture

Splits in the choroid and Bruch's membrane are seen as pale subretinal streaks, often concentric with the disc. They may be complicated by subretinal neovascular membrane formation, subretinal oedema, accumulation of subretinal hard exudate, or haemorrhage.

Blowout fracture

The bones of the floor and medial wall of the orbit (the roof of the maxillary antrum and the wall of the ethmoid sinus, respectively) are thin. A blow to the eye (commonly a ball or a fist) raises the intraocular and intraorbital pressure. Usually the orbital floor (or occasionally the medial wall) gives way, resulting in a blowout fracture rather than scleral rupture.

The symptoms, signs and complications of blowout are caused by the defect between orbit and antrum, and herniation of orbital tissues through the fracture.

Symptoms and signs

- Diplopia   Usually restriction of elevation of the affected eye, due to entrapment of the inferior intermuscular septum or inferior rectus, in the fracture. Depression is restricted because of trauma to inferior rectus.
- Epistaxis.
- Periocular surgical emphysema
  Air passes from the nasopharynx through the antrum and into the orbit following nose-blowing.
- Enophthalmos   The eye is retracted, as orbital tissue herniates into the antrum.
- Paraesthesia   The infraorbital nerve is usually damaged in blowout fracture of the orbital floor, causing paraesthesia in its distribution (the cheek and the upper incisor)
- X-ray   Opacification in the maxillary antrum caused by blood, and a 'hanging drop' from the orbital floor, indicating depressed fracture with downward herniation of orbital tissue.

Management

- Assess the eye for ocular injury.
- Measure enophthalmos with an exophthalmometer.
- Record eye movements on a Hess chart.
- Give antibiotics to prevent orbital infection due to contamination from the nose and sinuses.

Manage orbital blowout with minor degrees of tissue prolapse conservatively; document the stabilization of eye movements using serial Hess charts. Treat residual ocular motility disorder by appropriate elective muscle surgery as a secondary planned procedure.

Early surgical repair (3–10 days) is indicated if there is considerable tissue prolapse causing marked enophthalmos and restriction of movement. Orbital tissues are reduced surgically from the antrum, and the bony defect is supported with a silastic sheet introduced below the orbital periosteum.

Penetrating trauma

A perforating eye injury may be complicated by infection and intraocular tissue disruption, causing haemorrhage, inflammation, cataract, retinal detachment, sympathetic ophthalmitis, and phthisis. It is important to suspect perforation if the history or symptoms suggest it is a possibility, and to look carefully for signs of perforation, if necessary exploring beneath injured conjunctiva.

The prognosis of a perforated eye is always guarded. The patient should be warned of the serious nature of the injury, and the threat to sight. Properly managed, many perforated eyes recover well and retain good vision.

Signs of perforation

Direct inspection in focal illumination reveals corneal and anterior scleral perforation.

Aqueous leak is shown by fluorescein staining and blue light illumination at the slit-lamp (Siedel's test), shallow or flat anterior chamber, or reduced IOP.

Dark tissue presenting through cornea or sclera indicates uveal prolapse (iris or ciliary body) through a perforation. Vitreous may prolapse through a more posterior wound.

Pupil deformation is caused by prolapse of peripheral iris through a wound.

Loss of, or opacification in, the red pupil reflex, or hyphaema, may indicate intraocular disruption.

IOFB may be revealed radiographically.

Management

Immediately

Assess and stabilize the injury. Carry out as full an ophthalmological examination as is practicable, without delay, at the slit-lamp or on a couch. It is important to record visual acuities, pupil reactions, and the findings on dilated fundus examination, since progressive haemorrhage or rapid lens opacification may make later fundus examination impossible.

Clean the eye and remove foreign matter. Give topical antibiotics and protect the eye with a shield. Arrange surgical repair as soon as the patient is ready for anaesthesia. At primary surgery, retained objects are removed, non-viable tissue is excised, and viable tissue is reposited; perforations are repaired with prolene, dacron, or 8.0 virgin silk to sclera, and 10.0 nylon or prolene to cornea. Primary repair is carried out on all injuries; enucleation should always be a secondary procedure, undertaken only with the patient's express consent if the eye has no visual prognosis.

Repair of penetrating ocular trauma requires general anaesthesia. The risk of retrobulbar haemorrhage, followed by uncontrollable expulsion of the ocular contents through the perforation, contraindicates retrobulbar anaesthesia.

Corneal laceration and perforation

Perforating intracorneal foreign bodies must be removed with care, lest the anterior chamber collapses during removal, impaling the lens. Lacerated cornea is debrided and repaired under the operating microscope using 10.0 prolene, while the anterior chamber is maintained with viscoelastic through a paracentesis.

IOFB

Any perforating injury which may conceivably be associated with IOFB must be X-rayed. Symptoms and signs may be minimal.

Large IOFBs cause considerable trauma to the eye and orbit on impact; the possibility of IOFB is evident from the history and examination. Assessment includes X-ray, ultrasound, and CT.

Small IOFBs may cause minimal or occult external signs, and must be suspected from the history. High-energy impact between brittle materials causes small high velocity fragments to break off; these often cause minimal immediate symptoms or signs, and present the greatest risk of missed IOFB. Hammering a metal object, particularly a cold chisel or masonry nail, is a notorious source of a small IOFB which escapes detection.

Symptoms

There may have been a foreign body sensation on impact, followed by little or no discomfort. Vision may be normal initially, but is progressively impaired by haemorrhage, development of cataract, or inflammation. Developing uveitis causes gradually increasing discomfort over hours or days, and photophobia.

Endophthalmitis causes severe visual impairment delayed by hours or days; the visual loss caused by chemical toxicity (iron or copper) from metallic IOFB, is a late complication.

Signs

The entry wound may be visible at the slit-lamp: corneal wounds are best seen with scleral scatter or retroillumination; fluorescein staining shows an epithelial defect at entry site, which may leak (Siedel positive) or be self-sealing. A scleral entry site is generally covered by localized conjunctival injury, which may obscure the perforation.

Lens perforation is seen on dilated examination as an opacity in the red pupil reflex, or on retroilluminated slit-lamp examination.

Dilated fundus examination shows posterior segment damage, haemorrhage, or IOFB. Full dilated posterior segment examination must be part of the initial assessment of such injuries, in case rapidly progressive cataract formation makes later fundus examination impossible.

X-rays and localization

X-rays are taken in elevation and depression, so that any opacity within the orbit can be identified as moving with the eye (intraocular), or not (extraocular). The position of an IOFB can be approximately localized from lateral X-rays. A pre-equatorial foreign body moves in the same direction as the eye's vertical movement, while a post-equatorial foreign body moves in the opposite direction.

CT examination has superseded precise localization using a scleral ring and trigonometric analysis of X-ray plates; this method remains useful when CT is unavailable.

Ultrasound (B-mode) is useful in localizing the position of an IOFB within the eye.

Surgical management

An IOFB must be removed surgically, using vitrectomy techniques or the electromagnet. Non-magnetizable and organic IOFB must be removed directly, or by pars plana vitrectomy.

Give topical and systematic antibiotics following initial assessment. Post-operatively give topical steroids and mydriatics to suppress uveitis, and continue antibiotics.

Complications

1. *Infection*. Infection is unusual following high velocity metallic IOFB, but is extremely likely with an organic IOFB (e.g. wood splinter).

2. *Uveitis*.

3. *Retinal detachment*. A retinal tear sustained during injury may lead to early retinal detachment, shown by ultrasound scan if cataract or posterior segment haemorrhage obscures ophthalmoscopic view.

Traction detachment, caused by contraction of retinal scars, occurs after a delay of weeks or months, in association with proliferative vitreoretinopathy.

4. *Siderosis*. Retained ferrous IOFB causes irreversible direct retinal toxicity, and consequent visual loss, accompanied by heterochromia (green discoloration of the iris).

5. *Chalcosis*. Large copper foreign bodies release sufficient copper to cause early endophthalmitis. Smaller quantities of copper cause delayed cataract formation, and sometimes retinal detachment.

6. *Phthisis*. Severe intraocular disruption, especially involving the ciliary body or producing cyclitic membrane and traction, may led to progressive collapse and shrinkage of the eyeball.

Sympathetic ophthalmitis

Sympathetic is a chronic uveitis involving both the injured and the normal eye, following perforating injury involving uveal and retinal disruption. It has an autoimmune basis, probably due to exposure of lymphocytes to retinal antigens.

The condition presents from months to years following initial trauma, with signs of plastic or granulomatous uveitis in both eyes accompanied by creamy subretinal plaques (Dalen–Fuchs nodules).

Immediate accurate repair of perforating injuries, and control of inflammation with topical steroids, has reduced the incidence of sympathetic ophthalmitis. Once established, it presents a constant threat to the sympathizing eye, which must be treated with steroids and monitored indefinitely. The possibility that sympathetic ophthalmitis may develop in the fellow eye is one of the factors which must be taken into account when considering enucleation a blind eye following serious trauma.

Recommended further reading

Deutsch, T.A. and Feller, O.B. (1985). *Paton and Goldberg's management of ocular injuries*, 2nd edn. W. B. Saunders, Philadelphia.

Eagling, E.M. and Roper-Hall, M.J. (1986). *Eye injuries: an illustrated guide*. Butterworths, London.

Shingleton, B.J., Hersh, P.S., and Kenyon, K.R. (1991). *Eye trauma*. Mosby, St Louis.

12

The management of surgical patients

The regimens for management of surgical patients given below are a guide; details vary among units and between ophthalmologists. It is important to be familiar with individual preferences for steroid, antibiotic, or mydriatic preparations for routine use, and for preoperative and postoperative regimens, when ordering treatment.

Clerking

Ophthalmic clerking should ensure that:

1. The patient's general medical condition is understood and suitably managed.
2. The patient is fit for the proposed surgery and anaesthesia.
3. The results of a full preoperative eye examination are recorded, including: visual acuities; pupil reactions; intraocular pressure (IOP); biometry for cataract surgical patients; recent visual field assessment for glaucoma patients; detachment chart for vitreoretinal surgical patients.
4. The patient understands the purpose, nature, and possible complications of the proposed surgery, and that the eye for operation is agreed and clearly recorded in the notes.

History

Record the presenting complaint and its duration, past ocular history, and family history of eye trouble. Note also general medical conditions and their treatment.

Examination

General examination

Chest and cardiovascular system (CVS) to ensure fitness for surgery and anaesthesia. A previously unrecognized medical disorder should be treated or referred as appropriate.

Eye examination

Examine and record:

- visual acuities (aided and unaided), pupil responses for signs of external

inflammation (especially blepharitis and dacryocystitis before elective intra-ocular surgery);
- anterior segments at the slit-lamp, and measure IOPs;
- the fundi, after dilation;
- refraction, if unaided visual acuity is unaccountably poor;
- biometry, visual fields, gonioscopy, ultrasound, if appropriate.

Investigations

Routine investigation for general anaesthesia should be ordered according to local practice: an electrocardiogram is usually required by the anaesthetist for older patients and those with a history of cardiovascular disease; chest X-ray, haemoglobin, and biochemistry may not be necessary routinely.

Patients planned for surgery under local anaesthetic need routine medical examination, and signs of extraocular disease should be investigated appropriately.

Endophthalmitis

Endophthalmitis is a serious, sight-threatening ocular infection which may be caused by a wide range of pathogens. It is most commonly a complication of elective intraocular surgery, but may arise following trauma, and is occasionally endogenous.

The commonest infecting agents are:

Post-surgical   coagulase negative staphylococcus
staphylococcus aureus
streptococcus
other Gram positive organisms, eg propionibacterium
Gram negative organisms
fungi, eg candida and aspergillus

Traumatic   bacillus spp
coagulase negative staphylococcus
streptococcus
Gram negative organisms
fungi

Endogenous   candida spp
aspergillus spp

Almost any organism may occasionally cause intraocular infection, including anaerobes, spirochaetales, mycobacteria, viruses, and parasites.

Investigation

When endophthalmitis is suspected collect the following specimens:

1. Conjunctival swabs.
2. Swab from any wound, abscess or fistula, if present.

3. Anterior chamber tap.
4. Vitreous biopsy (using vitrectomy instrumentation through the pars plana).
5. Foreign body, if present.

The swabs should be plated immediately whenever possible, or alternatively placed in charcoal transport media, and fluids and the vitreous specimen submitted to the laboratory in a capped syringe or in a sterile universal container, marked 'endophthalmitis — urgent'. It is good practice to discuss suspected cases of endophthalmitis with the microbiologist before sending specimens, in order that arrangements may be made for immediate Gram stain and culture.

Management

Before diagnosis confirmed

Postoperative
Consider all serious postoperative inflammation as potentially infective, particularly if there is significant or increasing fibrin in the anterior chamber, or if there are cells in the anterior vitreous. If in doubt give intensive topical dexamethasone 0.1% for 6–12 hours, and re-assess. Eyes which deteriorate during, or relapse after this period should be treated as infected.

Trauma
Use prophylactic ciprofloxacin 200mg bd before primary repair.

Once diagnosis confirmed

Anti-inflammatory
Consider the use of high-dose oral steroid in severe cases (prednisolone 40–80 mg orally). Give atropine 1% drops tds to ensure maximum cycloplegia and mydriasis.

Antibiotic
Give a broad spectrum regimen initially, making appropriate modifications subsequently according to the results of culture and sensitivity.

Topical

Topical agents do not penetrate well into aqueous, with the exception of quinolones. Topical agents are not usually very effective, and should therefore not be relied upon as the sole mode of treatment in endophthalmitis. In mild cases, where the infection is confined to the anterior segment, use intensive(hourly drops) ofloxacin 0.3% until culture results are available.

Intravitreal

Initial empirical therapy: ceftazidime 2 mg plus vancomycin 2 mg, both in 0.1 ml under direct visual control into mid-vitreous.

Systemic

Penetration of antibiotics other than chloramphenicol, and possibly cipro-floxacin, into the eye is unreliable. However, in order to reduce the diffusion gradient of intraocular antibiotic out of the eye, and thereby to retain effective concentrations in the ocular tissues, the antibiotics given intravitreally should also be given systemically, ie:

> ceftazidime 2g tds
> vancomycin 1g bd, or a dose adjusted for renal function

Continuation of treatment

If no aetiological diagnosis is made, the broad spectrum regimen should be continued. Systemic antibiotics should be given for two weeks, and intravitreal antibiotic doses should be repeated every four days for up to two weeks, according to clinical response. A trough serum vancomycin level should be measured just before the third dose, and thereafter repeated twice-weekly while the treatment continues.

When an aetiological diagnosis has been reached, one of the above agents may be discontinued, and treatment continued with the other, as appropriate:

> Gram positive organisms: continue vancomycin
> Gram negative organisms: continue ceftazidime

These treatment outlines may require modification in the light of sensitivities of the infecting organism, and clinical response.

Unusual organisms (eg fungi, mycobacteria, anaerobes) require special treatment to be agreed on an individual patient basis between ophthalmologist and microbiologist.

Surgical treatment

In the presence of severe infection, pathogens of very high virulence (eg pseudomonas aeruginosa, Bacillus cereus, Staphylococcus aureus), a RAPD (indicating serious posterior segment damage), or intraocular foreign body, and in chronic cases, vitrectomy should be considered.

Cataract surgery

Indications

Cataract surgery is indicated when lens opacities are responsible for reduction in visual acuity sufficient to cause significant inconvenience. In general the patient indicates at what stage surgery is necessary, and the ophthalmologist helps balance the equation between likely benefits and potential complications.

Preoperative assessment

Exclude other causes of reduced acuity, and estimate the effect of lens opacities on visual function. Inspect for signs of external infection (conjunctivitis, blepharitis, dacryocystitis); elective surgery should never be undertaken in an infected eye. Take swabs, give appropriate antibiotics, and arrange re-admission when the infection has been eliminated.

Biometry

Estimate the appropriate intraocular lens (IOL) power preoperatively.

- Measure the radius of corneal curvature (K) and axial length (AL) using keratometry and ultrasound A-scan.
- Compute the IOL power by calculation (usually an automatic function within the A-scan instrument); ensure that the A-constant (defined by the type of IOL) is correctly entered. Postoperative refraction is generally aimed to be emmetropia or 1D myopia, but if the other eye is highly ametropic it may be necessary to calculate for a similar degree of ametropia in order to avoid aniseikonic diplopia.

Postoperative management

Remove the dressing on the morning of the first postoperative day, and inspect for discharge, wound integrity, corneal clarity, anterior chamber depth and clarity, pupil shape, and IOL position. Measure intraocular pressure (IOP) if the cornea is cloudy. Examine the anterior vitreous for cells, and the disc and macula with the indirect ophthalmoscope.

Routine postoperative topical medication (for 2 weeks, or until the eye is quiet):

- topical steroid (betamethasone, prednisolone or dexamethasone q.d.s.)
- mydriatic (cyclopentolate 1 per cent b.d.)
- (antibiotic)

Complications

Wound gape or dehiscence, iris prolapse
Wounds which are inadequately closed require resuturing without delay. Small leaks (Siedel positive but wound otherwise secure) often become watertight without intervention in a few days.

Postoperative uveitis
A degree of anterior uveitis inevitably follows cataract surgery, especially following IOL implantation. It is more marked in diabetics, following incomplete aspiration of lens cortex, and following posterior capsule rupture. Routine steroid and mydriatic postoperative drops are usually adequate, but need to be more intensive if inflammation is more severe.

Corneal oedema
Cloudy cornea following anterior segment surgery indicates endothelial decompensation, as a result of:

1. Raised IOP (idiopathic, uveitis, or retained viscoelastic material).
2. Poor endothelial function: (a) surgical trauma to the endothelium; (b) lens–endothelial touch (anterior chamber IOLs); (c) endothelial dystrophy.

Give acetazolamide (250 mg s.r. b.d.) to reduce IOP, and treat uveitis with adequate topical steroids. Treatment can usually be reduced in a few days. If endothelial dysfunction is severe and irreversible, bullous keratopathy may follow.

Cystoid macular oedema (CMO)
Causes unexpectedly poor postoperative acuity in the presence of clear media. Diagnosis is by 78D lens examination at the slit-lamp, and fluorescein angiography. CMO is commoner following intracapsular than extracapsular (ECCE) cataract extraction or phacoemulsification, and in ECCE is commoner following vitreous loss. Treatment with indomethacin, acetazolamide, or periocular steroid injection is sometimes recommended, but CMO often resolves spontaneously.

Posterior capsule opacification
Gradual deterioration in acuity beginning weeks or months after cataract surgery. Opacification, due to lens epithelial proliferation, is visible at the slit-lamp and obscures fundus detail. Treat by YAG capsulotomy, using a contact lens with a dilated pupil.

Loose or degenerating sutures
Loose sutures cause irritation, accumulate mucus and stimulate corneal vascularization. They should be removed under topical anaesthesia at the slit-lamp.

Refractive correction
Refract the eye at each postoperative visit. High cylindrical errors are caused by sutures which are too tight or too loose. A tight suture induces astigmatism corrected by a +cylinder whose axis lies in line with the suture. Reduce corneal astigmatism before ordering the spectacle correction by dividing this suture, or the entire continuous suture, not sooner than 8 weeks postoperatively. Order glasses after corneal astigmatism has stabilized (usually 2 months' postoperatively).

Secondary IOL implantation

Indications
Intolerance of aphakia or difficulty with contact lens, especially if the other eye has good phakic or pseudophakic vision.

Preoperative assessment

As for cataract extraction. Secondary IOLs are usually placed in the anterior chamber; it is important to use the appropriate A-constant and aphakic measuring mode when computing IOL power. Constrict the pupil preoperatively with pilocarpine.

Glaucoma surgery

The appropriate surgical procedure depends on the aetiology of glaucoma in any individual case, and particularly on the status of the drainage angle. The considerations which determine management of glaucoma are described more fully in Chapter 5.

Trabeculectomy creates a fistula between the anterior chamber and the subconjunctival space, by the excision of a small segment of the trabecular meshwork beneath a scleral flap. It is used to shunt aqueous when drainage through the trabecular meshwork is reduced (in primary open angle glaucoma (POAG), and chronic angle closure glaucoma).

Peripheral iridectomy or iridotomy creates an alternative channel for the circulation of aqueous from the posterior to the anterior chamber in narrow angle and acute angle closure glaucoma, and relieves pupil block in secondary glaucoma.

Argon laser trabeculoplasty has a limited place, supplementing medical treatment when trabeculectomy is not possible or contraindicated. It may effect a modest reduction in IOP in these cases, but is generally not a satisfactory alternative to definitive drainage surgery, and its effect often reduces over 1–5 years. Fifty to 100 small high power burns (50 μm × 600–1000 mW × 0.1 s) are placed around 180° of mid-anterior trabecular meshwork.

Plate and tube drainage explants are used in glaucoma which has proved resistant to conventional drainage surgery, or in which such procedures are likely to fail. Rubeotic glaucoma is resistant to conventional drainage surgery because the trabeculectomy becomes sealed by fibrovascular proliferation. The Molteno tube, and other devices, drain the anterior chamber through an indwelling silicone tube connected to a plate sutured externally to the sclera.

Cyclocryotherapy and cyclodialysis (cryoablation or detachment of a segment of the ciliary body) are sometimes used to reduce IOP in an eye where conventional surgery has repeatedly failed or is impossible. The results of such procedures are generally less predictable than those of drainage procedures, but cyclocryotherapy has a place in the management of some glaucomas which occur following complicated vitreoretinal surgical disorders and their surgery.

Indications for glaucoma surgery

Trabeculectomy is increasingly widely considered as a first-line management option in established POAG. More traditionally, surgery is considered when

IOP is inadequately controlled on medical treatment, in the presence of progressive glaucomatous field loss.

Trabeculectomy

Preoperative assessment

Ensure that recent or preoperative visual fields are available, confirming progressive glaucomatous loss. Explain to the patient that surgery is not intended to improve vision, but to prevent it from further deterioration, and that it may become transiently worse (due to hyphaema or flat anterior chamber) immediately after surgery.

Postoperative management

Examine at the slit-lamp for hyphaema, uveitis, cornea and lens clarity, anterior chamber depth, aqueous leak from beneath the conjunctival margin at the bleb, and IOP. Order routine postoperative topical therapy (steroid and mydriatic).

Complications

Hyphaema

Transient hyphaema following trabeculectomy is common; if the anterior chamber is formed, hyphaema usually resorbs in a few days. Total hyphaema with elevated IOP requires intensive dilation to prevent pupil block. Rarely, surgical evacuation may be necessary.

Flat anterior chamber

Postoperative shallowing or flattening of the anterior chamber is a common complication of drainage surgery. It usually resolves without intervention, but its cause must be identified and treated. Check for:

1. Aqueous leak beneath the conjunctival flap by Siedel test (stain the tear film with fluorescein; a green dribble of non-staining aqueous shows the site of a leak, when viewed under blue illumination).
2. Choroidal effusion, using the indirect ophthalmoscope through dilated pupil. Effusions appear as convex dome-shaped dark swellings in the periphery of the fundus, of which the anterior limit cannot be seen. They are usually located inferonasally, inferolaterally, or both.

Treat flat postoperative anterior chamber with intensive cycloplegia, using phenylephrine and atropine, and apply a firm dressing pad for 24 h periods until the anterior chamber deepens. If there is accompanying choroidal effusion, acetazolamide (500 mg, b.d. orally) may help, by reducing outflow through the uveoscleral channels, which is facilitated by the choroidal effusion.

If a completely flat anterior chamber fails to re-form after a week, further surgical intervention must be considered. Subchoroidal fluid is drained through a pars plana sclerotomy, and the anterior chamber is reformed using air introduced through a surgical cyclodialysis cleft originating at the sclerotomy.

Drainage failure
Failure of trabeculectomy to control the IOP postoperatively is due to closure of the drainage fistula by fibrosis, and is often accompanied by encystment of the bleb. Early drainage failure (during the first 3 weeks following surgery) can often be reversed by digital massage of the bleb, either through the closed upper lid, or directly to the anaesthetized conjunctiva overlying the scleral trapdoor, using a cotton wool bud. Late drainage failure can only be addressed by re-opening the scleral flap and formal revision of the trabeculectomy, or by undertaking a new trabeculectomy in a fresh meridian of the limbus. Such second procedures are often supplemented by subconjunctival 5-fluorouracil injections to inhibit postoperative fibrosis.

Trabeculectomy fails more commonly in eyes which are inflamed or undergoing proliferation, especially rubeosis, and in negroes.

Cataract
Cataract formation after trabeculectomy is often delayed, and occurs more commonly in eyes which have undergone postoperative complications.

Retinal detachment surgery

Indications

Rhegmatogenous retinal detachment requires surgical repair. Traction detachment is repaired:

1. if the development of a retinal break converts it to a rhegmatogenous detachment;
2. if the detachment is progressive;
3. if vision is reduced by macular involvement.

The aim of surgery for rhegmatogenous detachment is to close and seal the hole, to prevent recruitment of subretinal fluid into the subretinal space. Traction detachment is treated by vitrectomy, removal of epiretinal membranes by peeling (delamination) and segmentation, supplemented if necessary by internal tamponade with silicone oil or gas.

Preoperative assessment

Chart the shape and extent of the detachment, and the positions of retinal breaks (red for attached, blue for detached retina) using the indirect ophthalmoscope. Examine the fellow eye equally carefully, since the factors predisposing to retinal detachment are bilateral, and asymptomatic breaks require prophylactic cryotherapy at the time of surgery.

Postoperative management

Keep the pupil dilated with atropine. Postural nursing may be necessary if intraocular gas has been used to effect internal tamponade, in order to keep the break uppermost, and thereby to maximize the effect of the gas bubble in tamponading the break. If subretinal fluid has not been drained surgically, it resorbs spontaneously providing the breaks have been closed completely.

Complications

Failed retinal reattachment
Persistent detachment is caused by failure to close the break or breaks. This may be due to inadequate, inaccurate, or inappropriate buckling, missed breaks, or distorted breaks or retinal shortening due to epiretinal membrane formation.

Choroidal and vitreous haemorrhage
Subretinal fluid drainage may be complicated by choroidal haemorrhage into the subretinal space. This settles without treatment, but may compromise the final visual acuity if it involves the macula. The risk of bleeding at the time of subretinal fluid drainage is minimized by maintaining the IOP throughout the procedure.

Plomb infection and extrusion
Pain, inflammation, and discharge following explant surgery suggest plomb infection. The site of the plomb should be examined, and a broad spectrum antibiotic given; infected plombs will extrude spontaneously, or require surgical removal. A plomb which presents through the conjunctiva should be removed. Plomb removal more than 6 months following successful reattachment is seldom followed by redetachment.

Anterior segment ischaemia
Encircling procedures are occasionally complicated by anterior segment ischaemia, which presents as intense painful anterior uveitis. It is important not to overtighten the encirclement, and to ensure that the IOP is not dangerously elevated by surgery, by checking the patency of the retinal vessels at the disc, which should be patent or pulsating.

Proliferative vitreoretinopathy (PVR)
Persistent retinal detachment in the presence of an open retinal break, especially when it follows failed surgical attempts at reattachment, leads to PVR. Epiretinal membrane formation leads to retinal stiffening and shortening, and distortion of the break. Reattachment by conventional surgical means is impossible due to reduced retinal mobility and vitrectomy techniques are necessary.

Dacryocystorhinostomy (DCR)

Tear drainage obstruction caused by occlusion of the lacrimal sac or nasolacrimal duct follows recurrent or chronic infection, either of the sac or the exit of the duct beneath the inferior turbinate. DCR creates a surgical fistula between the sac and the nasopharynx, through the wall of the lacrimal fossa to enter the nasopharynx beneath the middle turbinate.

Indications

Recurrent dacryocystitis, or watering due to sac or nasolacrimal duct obstruction, demonstrated by syringing, which causes significant distress. DCR requires general anaesthesia, sometimes using hypotensive techniques and vasoconstrictors, and cardiovascular disorder therefore generally contraindicates DCR surgery.

Preoperative assessment

Identify the site of the obstruction by syringing the tear ducts. Treat dacryocystitis with antibiotics before surgery. Dacryocystography (radiography using contrast injected into the lacrimal system to identify site of stenosis or obstruction) is sometimes helpful. Dacryocystography may identify a lacrimal sac tumour, but as the procedure takes place at an unphysiologically high hydraulic pressure, functional obstruction is not incompatible with radiological patency

Postoperative management

Apply a pressure bandage at the end of the operation to reduce bleeding, leaving it in place until the following day. Persistent haemorrhage is uncommon, and presents as postoperative epistaxis. Chart pulse and blood pressure observations, and give intravenous fluids or blood transfusion if necessary. Remove skin sutures 1 week postoperatively. Leave the silastic tube (O'Donoghue or Crawford) in place for about 6 months, to act as a splint for mucosal repair in the DCR. Remove it by dividing the loop in the inner canthus; the tube is expelled when the patient blows his nose.

Complications

Tube prolapse
This usually follows curious or unwitting manipulation by the patient, and is best avoided by warning the patient not to interfere with the tube. If the knot remains in the nasopharynx the tube can be pulled back down with forceps through a nasal speculum, after cocainization to shrink the inferior turbinate. If the knot has been pulled through the DCR into the sac, attempts to replace it are invariably unsuccessful, and it must be removed.

Failure of the DCR
If tubes have been used this is unusual. An inadequately sized bone resection is the commonest cause of failure. The fistula through the floor of the fossa should initially be some 2 cm diameter, but healing reduces it to much less than this, and may obliterate it completely.

Corneal graft (penetrating or lamellar keratoplasty)

Corneal grafting is undertaken for optical, and occasionally tectonic (to preserve the integrity of the eye if the cornea perforates due to ulceration, melting, or trauma) reasons. Penetrating keratoplasty is indicated if opacities involve the deep stroma, or if endothelial function is poor.

Lamellar keratoplasty preserves the host endothelium and is used in the presence of opacities confined to the superficial stroma in the presence of good endothelial function. Cataract extraction is combined with corneal graft if lens opacities coexist with corneal opacification.

Indications

Corneal opacity
Scarring following:

- keratitis,
- herpes simplex,
- bacterial corneal ulcer,
- interstitial keratitis,
- trauma.

Endothelial decompensation
- aphakic and pseudophakic bullous keratopathy,
- other post-surgical endothelial trauma,
- Fuchs' endothelial dystrophy.

Keratoconus
When contact lenses are no longer stable because of the steep cone.

Corneal stromal dystrophies
Particularly macular dystrophy (autosomal recessive).

Tectonic
Corneal perforation due to melting disorder, ulcer, or trauma.

Preoperative management

Recipient
The eye should be clean, without infection or inflammation, and IOP controlled preoperatively. HLA tissue typing is not routinely undertaken, but good tissue antigen match improves prognosis in high risk eyes. Miose the pupil pre-operatively with pilocarpine to protect the lens from surgical trauma; if ECCE is to be combined with corneal graft, dilate the pupil preoperatively.

Donor graft material
The following criteria are generally applied:

- HIV and hepatitis B negative.

- No CNS disease of possible prion protein aetiology (e.g. Jakob–Creutzfeldt).
- Donor under 65 years.
- Cause of donor death not malignant or infective disease.
- Collection of donor material as soon as practical after death, normally within 12 h, and then stored at 4°C.

Donor cornea may be used fresh, or cultured in nutrient medium. Fresh material must be used within 24–36 h, and provides optimal endothelial repopulation. Storage of donor cornea requires specialized techniques, and is undertaken by transplant laboratories. Intermediate storage in MK or K-sol media depletes donor material antigenicity, and reduces the risk of rejection; it also eliminates the risk of bacterial infection. For these reasons stored graft material is generally preferred for penetrating keratoplasty, especially in eyes in which the risk of rejection is high. Long-term storage by cryopreservation is not available clinically for whole cornea, but cryotechniques are appropriate for lamellar keratoplasty and epikeratophakia.

If corneal material from a suitable donor becomes available, but is not required for use as a fresh graft, the eyes should be accepted and forwarded to an eye bank for preservation of the corneas in culture medium, and distribution.

Postoperative management

Check for wound integrity with fluorescein, and monitor epithelial cover of the donor surface.

Postoperative control of inflammation and IOP is important. Treat with steroid drops to suppress inflammatory signs in the anterior chamber, and keep the pupil dilated for 4–8 weeks after surgery. Reduce IOP if necessary with topical beta-blocker or oral acetazolamide (NB Goldmann tonometry may be inaccurate following keratoplasty, as the corneal contour and compliance are altered; indentation tonometry, using tonopen or McKay–Marg, may be more accurate).

Leave sutures in place for 6–12 months. Loose sutures predispose to vascularization and rejection, and overtight sutures cause corneal astigmatism. In either case early suture removal may be necessary.

Complications

Loose wound
A loose wound, or a suture which fails or cuts through at the host or donor bite, may cause wound leak, flattening of the anterior chamber, iris incarceration, or iris prolapse. The pupil should be dilated intensively to prevent or reverse pupil block, and the graft re-sutured.

Failed re-epithelialization
If the donor epithelium has been removed, re-epithelialization by cells derived from the host limbus is usually complete within a week or two. Delayed epithelialization raises the risk of stromal ulceration, which can be reduced by fitting a bandage contact lens.

Glaucoma
Glaucoma following penetrating keratoplasty increases the risk of graft failure. It may be idiopathic, or due to pupil block or peripheral anterior synaechia. Temporary postoperative elevation of IOP due to retained viscoelastic material is common. It is controlled medically in the short term using acetazolamide, or surgically.

Astigmatism
A degree of distortion inevitably follows penetrating keratoplasty, but its magnitude depends on surgical technique. It is corrected with spectacles or hard contact lenses. Large degrees may be reduced by dividing the suture in the axis of the + cylinder.

Graft failure
Loss of clarity in the donor tissue suggests failure of a penetrating graft undertaken for optical reasons; such failure may be conveniently classified as early or delayed.

Early graft failure (within 1–5 days)
Persistent swelling of donor cornea by 50 per cent or more in thickness immediately following surgery suggests primary failure, due to poor initial endothelial cell function, or surgical trauma to the endothelium. Delayed recovery of endothelial function may occur during the first week. Regrafting may be undertaken within a week or two of primary failure in eyes which are otherwise healthy, but if there is inflammation or glaucoma a second graft is better delayed until these complications have been controlled medically, in order to reduce the risk of repeated failure.

Delayed
Progressive loss of corneal clarity following an initial clear period indicates delayed failure. This may be due to rejection, endothelial failure, recurrence of the original disease or a combination of these, and can occur within days of surgery, or be delayed by years.

Immunological rejection is facilitated by vascularization at the graft–host interface, by iris incarceration, by intraocular inflammation, and by raised IOP. Epithelium, stroma, or endothelium, or more than one layer, may be involved in rejection episodes, which are more common in high risk eyes (Table 12.1). The cardinal signs of rejection are anterior uveitis and a 'rejection' line of keratic precipitates on the endothelium with a zone of corneal decompensation behind it. Treat rejection episodes with intensive topical and oral steroids, and if necessary immunosuppressives; topical antiviral cover is also necessary in eyes grafted for herpes simplex keratitis. A proportion of grafts survives such episodes.

Delayed failure due to endothelial decompensation suggests either poor graft material, or surgical trauma.

Table 12.1   Eyes at high risk of graft rejection

Ocular inflammation at the time of surgery
Corneal neovascularization involving the graft/host junction
Previous failed grafts
Lid defects
Dry eye syndromes, especially pemphigoid
Uncontrolled glaucoma

Recurrence of the original disease occurs particularly in herpes simplex keratitis. Management of these eyes is particularly difficult since steroid treatment must be considered in addition to antiviral therapy, in order to minimize inflammation which may predispose to rejection.

Squint surgery

Most childhood squints are concomitant, with or without an accommodative element.
   Squints in adults may be:

- uncorrected or undercorrected childhood squints,
- consecutive squint following earlier surgery,
- neurological (paralytic),
- restrictive (inflammation, infiltration, or trauma).

Indications for surgery

- cosmetic
- functional   to correct diplopia
                to restore binocular vision
                to correct an abnormal head posture.

   Surgery is not undertaken in paralytic or restrictive squint until the angle has become stable.

Preoperative preparation

Orthoptic examination precedes the decision to operate, and measurements are repeated immediately before surgery. If it is not possible to resolve whether the ocular motor disorder is primarily due to restriction or weakness by pre-operative clinical assessment, duction tests may help. Active duction tests (to reveal muscle strength) must be carried out before surgery, while passive duction tests (to reveal restriction) are performed peroperatively.

Postoperative management

Assess the postoperative deviation and extraocular movements the day after surgery Give steroid drops or ointment for 2–4 weeks postoperatively, or until surgical inflammation has resolved. The correction stabilizes within a month or so of surgery.

Complications

The accuracy with which the angle of deviation is corrected depends partly on the preoperative binocular status. Eyes which have had good binocular function are more likely to achieve a satisfactory stable result. Eyes without binocular function lack the stability given by fusional vergence; undercorrection may lead to progressive reversion to the original deviation, while overcorrection may lead to consecutive deviation in the opposite direction.

Dehiscence of reinsertion
A large angle deviation after surgery, with failure of movement in the field of an operated muscle, suggests that the muscle has become detached from the eye. It must be surgically retrieved and resutured.

Stitch granuloma
A mass over the reinsertion of a muscle is caused by suture inflammation. It usually responds to topical steroid treatment and patience, but if persistent it may need to be excised.

Restriction
Late restriction of movement is caused by fibrotic adhesions, or excessive muscle recession, or excessive resection of the antagonist. Surgical manipulation of tissues and haemorrhage particularly predispose to adhesions.

Ptosis

Ptosis may be congenital or acquired, and is caused by physical, myogenic, or neurogenic factors.

Indications for surgery
- cosmetic
- functional Obstruction of the visual axis. It is important to consider the possible amblyogenic effect of visual deprivation in infants with ptosis.

Contraindications to ptosis surgery
- Duane's lid-retraction syndrome.
- Marcus–Gunn jaw-winking. Surgery is usually best avoided, though bilateral tarsal disinsertion and frontalis sling are sometimes performed.
- Corneal anaesthesia.
- Absent Bell's phenomenon.
- Dry eye.

Choice of surgical procedure

This depends on the aetiology and severity of the ptosis, and the levator function. The principles governing the choice of surgical procedure in ptosis surgery are given in Chapter 2, p. 18.

Preoperative assessment

- Exclude conditions which contraindicate ptosis surgery.
- Identify neurogenic (III palsy or Horner's syndrome) and myogenic (myasthenia, myopathy) causes of ptosis preoperatively.
- Measure the ptosis and levator function by holding a ruler vertically before the eye, while preventing effects of levator action on the lid by firm pressure over the brow.

Ptosis is measured as the difference in width between the palpebral fissures in the primary position. The normal upper lid covers the upper 2 mm of the cornea; in the assessment of bilateral ptosis, refer measurement to this normal lid height.

Levator function is measured as the lid margin excursion between maximum depression and maximal elevation.

Anaesthesia

General anaesthesia is necessary in children. Local anaesthesia is preferable in adults, especially in levator resection, when voluntary lid movement by the patient helps determine the correct length of muscle to be resected.

Postoperative management

Assess the adequacy of corneal cover by the upper lid on the first postoperative day. Remove a Frost suture if it has been used, and tie and trim temporary sutures if lid closure is satisfactory.

Examine and stain the cornea for signs of suture keratopathy (focal epithelial loss caused by an unburied knot). If this occurs, protect the cornea with a bandage contact lens, or remove the suture.

Initial assessment of the result of the operation is difficult because of the effect of postoperative tissue swelling.

Complications

The principal complications of ptosis surgery are undercorrection, overcorrection (which can be complicated by exposure keratopathy), and notching of the upper lid, which results from an improperly shaped tarso-aponeurotic resection or uneven reinsertion of levator. Suture keratopathy is sometimes a problem following the Fasanella tarso-levator resection, when an exposed knot causes corneal abrasion or ulceration.

When ptosis surgery is undertaken for cosmetic reasons it should be remembered that dissatisfaction with an imperfect result is likely to be greater in patients whose initial ptosis was least.

Enucleation, evisceration, and exenteration

Indications

Removal of the eye is necessary if it is blind and causes distress, or if it contains a potentially life-threatening tumour.

Evisceration is indicated if the eye is grossly infected, in order to avoid exposure of the subdural space of the optic nerve and the orbital veins, and thereby avoid possible backward spread of the infection.

Exenteration (removal of the entire contents of the orbit), combined with radiotherapy, is necessary if a malignant ocular tumour is complicated by extraocular spread, or for a malignant orbital tumour involving the eye.

Preoperative assessment

Review and confirm the indications for surgery to remove an eye. Routines for a joint staff opinion are established in many units, and should be followed. Discuss the nature of the proposed surgery explicitly with the patient, explaining how the socket will be managed after the eye has been removed.

The surgeon should mark the eye preoperatively, with the agreement of the patient.

Post operative management

Dress the socket with antibiotic ointment for a day or two before fitting a shell. This helps to maintain the fornices (which are important in stabilizing the definitive prosthesis) and should be removed, washed, and replaced daily. Prosthesis fitting is arranged 1–3 months after surgery, when the orbital tissues have healed and stabilized.

Complications

Recurrence of neoplasm must be excluded at postoperative reviews.

The post-enucleation socket syndrome describes the unsatisfactory cosmetic appearance caused by an ill-fitting artificial eye in an orbit with insufficient tissue bulk, or an insufficient mucosal lining. These problems may be treated surgically by autograft of, respectively, dermofat and mucous membrane.

Recommended further reading

Easty, D.L. (ed.) (1990). *Current ophthalmic surgery*. Baillière Tindall, London.

Rice, T.A., Michaels, R.G., Stark, W.J. (vol. eds), Dudley and Carter (Gen. ed.). (1984). *Rob and Smith's operative surgery. Ophthalmic surgery*, 4th edn. Butterworths, London.

Roper Hall, M.J. (1989). *Stallard's eye surgery*. 7th edn. Wright, London.

Waltman *et al.* (1988). *Surgery of the eye*. Churchill Livingstone, New York.

13

Optics and refraction

Optics and refraction

Visible light is electromagnetic radiation with a wavelength of between 480 and 800 nm, to which the retinal receptors respond by hyperpolarization of their cell membranes. Because vision depends on the presentation of a focused image of the external world to the retina, it is important to understand how the image is formed by the eye, and how defocus occurs, is measured and corrected.

Properties of light

The properties of light determine its velocity of conduction through transmitting media: space, air, glass, or the clear ocular tissues and fluids.

Velocity

The velocity of light in a vacuum is constant. It is reduced through transmitting media in proportion to their optical density. Because of this, a ray of light striking the interface between two transmitting media obliquely is refracted through an angle which depends on their optical densities.

Wavelength

Short wavelength light is refracted through a greater angle than long wavelength light. Because of this, white light is dispersed into its component spectral colours when it crosses an oblique interface between one transmitting medium and another. The wavelength of light determines colour sensation. Three distinct cone populations respond differentially to short, medium, and long wavelengths in the visible spectrum, producing the sensation of blue, green, and red, respectively. In practice only the longest and shortest wavelengths stimulate only one receptor population, and the sensations of intermediate colours are produced by the relative output in all three receptor populations.

Optics

Refraction

The deviation of a ray of light passing from one medium into another is called refraction. The magnitude of the angle of refraction r is determined by the angle of incidence i and the refractive indices of the two media, called n_1 and n_2, according to Snell's formula:

$$\frac{\sin i}{\sin r} = \frac{n_2}{n_1}.$$

If the first medium is air, whose refractive index may be considered to be 1, then

$$\frac{\sin i}{\sin r} = n_2 = \text{constant}.$$

Refraction at a plane surface produces a simple deviation in the path of light. If the interface is not plane but presents a curved surface to the incident light rays, then the angle of incidence varies, and therefore so also does the angle of refraction. A spherical surface brings the refracted rays to a point focus, and a cylindrical surface brings them to a line focus.

Some spectral dispersion occurs in refraction at both plane and curved surfaces, because the angle of refraction of shorter wavelengths is greater than that of longer wavelengths. The effect of this is to create an extended focus, with longer-wavelength rays meeting at a point more distant from the lens than short-wavelength rays. This is called chromatic aberration when it is produced by lenses, and is more marked in thicker lenses. It can be minimized by making a composite lens with a layer of high refractive index glass on one face. The effect is also used in the duochrome test (p. 254).

Diffusion and diffraction

Diffusion describes the scattering of rays caused by opacities or discontinuities in a transmitting or refracting medium. Diffusion occurs clinically in cataract.

Diffraction describes the effect of regular discontinuities in a refracting medium, which give rise to an array of secondary point or line sources of light. The interaction of rays of light emerging from these secondary point or line sources is called interference.

Lenses

A convex lens (Fig. 13.1) brings parallel rays of light to a point focus posterior to the lens. A concave lens (Fig. 13.2) diverges rays of light as if from an imaginary (virtual) focus anterior to the lens.

Thin lenses

'Thin lens' theory describes the theoretical behaviour of light rays through simple lenses, in which the total power of the lens is equal to the sum of the

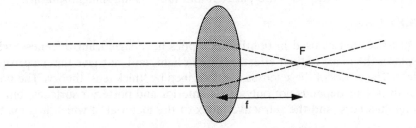

Fig. 13.1   The path of light rays through a convex (plus) lens. Parallel rays are brought to a focus F, at f cm from the centre of the lens. The power of this lens is $+1/f$ dioptres.

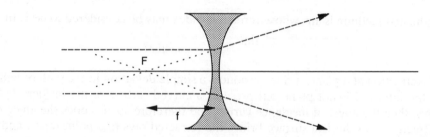

Fig. 13.2   The path of light rays through a concave (minus) lens. Parallel rays diverge from a virtual focus F, at $-f$ cm from the centre of the lens. The power of this lens is $-1/f$ dioptres.

powers of the two (anterior and posterior) refracting surfaces, and deviation occurs at a plane which is located in the centre of the lens. The focal length of a thin lens is the distance from its optical centre to its focal point. The power of the lens (expressed in dioptres) is the reciprocal of its focal length expressed in metres. The focal length and power of a lens may be defined according to real or virtual focal points; by convention the power of a convex, or converging, lens is given a plus sign, while a concave, or diverging lens has minus power.

Thin lens $F = F1 + F2$
(F = total power; $F1$ = anterior surface power; $F2$ = posterior surface power)

Lens systems

When two or more lenses are arranged as a system, their effect on the path of rays of light may be replaced by a single 'equivalent' thin lens. However, the planes at which deviation occurs are not coincident with the centre of the equivalent lens, but outside it at the *principal planes* of the system. The position at which the equivalent lens must be placed to replicate the back vertex properties of the lens system is called the *second principal plane*, while the plane at which it must be placed to replicate the front vertex properties of the system is called the *first principal plane*. The principal planes cross the axis at the *principal points*. The principal planes (Fig. 13.3) are conjugate planes between which no deviation occurs (i.e. rays are paraxial and there is unit magnification).

Thick lenses

In practice, lenses used in ophthalmic optics have significant thickness, which displaces the plane of their effect on rays of light, and may give them a prismatic effect. The optics of these lenses are described by 'thick lens' theory. The power of a thick lens depends not only on its anterior and posterior surfaces, but also on its thickness, and the refractive index of the material of which it is made.

Thick lens $F = F1 + F2 - dF1F2$
d = lens thickness.

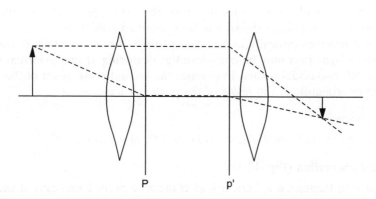

Fig. 13.3   Light rays passing through a lens system. P = first principal plane; p' = second principal plane.

A thick lens may be considered as a special kind of lens system, in which two refracting surfaces are separated by glass; this intervening thickness of glass has the same effect as would a (greater) intervening thickness of air. Fig. 13.4 shows the path of rays of light through a thick lens. Note the behaviour of rays at the principal planes (cf. a lens system), and that rays entering the system towards the *first nodal point* leave as though from the *second nodal point* with their direction of travel unchanged. The focal length of a thick lens is, in practice, measured from the posterior vertex of the lens (the posterior vertex focal length) or from its anterior vertex (the anterior vertex focal length).

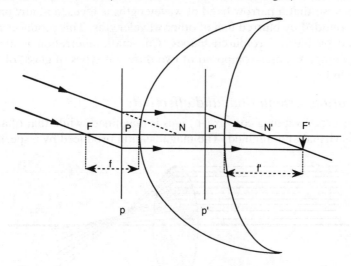

Fig. 13.4   Light rays passing through a thick lens. F = anterior focal point; F' = posterior focal point; f = anterior vertex focal length; f' = posterior vertex focal length; p = first principal plane; p' = second principal plane; P = first principal point; P' = second principal point; N = first nodal point; N' = second nodal point.

The anterior and posterior focal points, the principal points and the nodal points together constitute the six *cardinal points* of a thick lens.

The eye behaves optically as a system of thick lenses, in which deviation in the path of light rays may be considered as occurring at two principal planes, and through two nodal points. In practice the second nodal point of the human eye is approximately at the plane of the posterior lens capsule.

Aberrations

The performance of simple lenses is limited by aberrations.

Spherical aberration (Fig. 13.5)

Rays passing through a spherical lens come to a point focus only if they pass through its most central part (i.e. if it has a small aperture). An extended focus is produced from a larger aperture, since more peripheral zones of the lens have a steeper curve, which refracts the rays through a larger angle than the central zone.

Spherical aberration is avoided by reducing the effective aperture, and designing aspheric (e.g. parabolic) lenses.

Distortion of oblique rays and coma (Fig. 13.6)

Only axial rays converge at a point focus; those striking the anterior face of a lens at an angle to its axis meet an oblique refracting surface, and emerge to form a focus which is elongated in the line of obliquity.

Chromatic aberration (Fig. 13.7)

The greater angle of refraction of short wavelengths causes spectral separation of the focus, so that a narrow band of wavelengths is focused at any one plane, and is surrounded by blurred foci of other wavelengths. This produces an image surrounded by blurred coloured haloes. Chromatic aberration is avoided by designing complex lenses composed of two different types of glass, of different refractive index.

Magnification, orientation, and effectivity

The image produced by a convex (+) lens is magnified, while that of a concave (−) lens is virtual and minified. The magnification produced by a spectacle lens

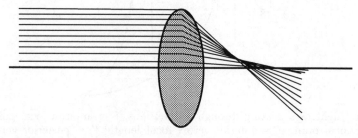

Fig. 13.5 Spherical aberration. Paraxial rays are refracted through a smaller angle than those striking the periphery of the lens.

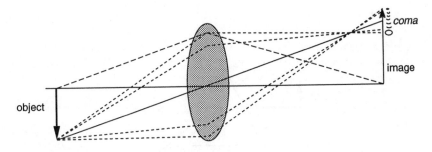

Fig. 13.6 Distortion of oblique rays. Oblique rays passing through different zones of the lens are subject to different degrees of magnification, producing a 'coma' (cf. comet's tail).

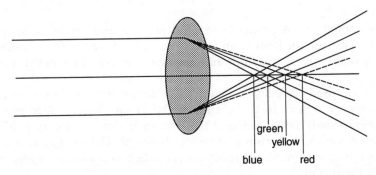

Fig. 13.7 Chromatic aberration. Short wavelength light is refracted through a greater angle than longer wavelengths, causing dispersion of the emerging rays, with the blue image nearer to the lens than the red image.

depends upon its power and the distance from its posterior surface (the 'back vertex') to the cornea (the 'back vertex distance', or BVD, of the lens). The greater the BVD, the greater the lens' effectivity. This effect leads to the formation of images of different sizes (aniseikonia) on the two retinas if there is a large difference between the refracting power of the two eyes (anisometropia), such as in unilateral aphakia. The problems of aniseikonic diplopia in unilateral aphakia are completely overcome by correcting the anisometropia with an intraocular lens placed in the position of the physiological lens, where its effectivity is unchanged. The effectivity of contact lenses (BVD = 0) is less than that of spectacle lenses, and they therefore produce less magnification, and a degree of aniseikonia which is normally tolerated without diplopia.

Prisms

A prism deviates the path of light rays through an angle which is determined by the angle of its apex; the image seen through a prism is deviated towards its apex (Fig. 13.8). Prisms used in ophthalmic practice are measured in 'prism

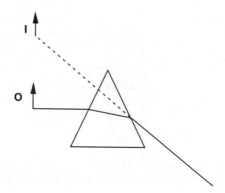

Fig. 13.8   The deviation produced by a prism.

dioptres', noted 'Δ'. A prism of strength 1 prism dioptre produces an apparent linear displacement of 1 cm of an object situated 1 m away. The orientation of prisms is defined by the position of their base (base-up, base-down, base-out, base-in).

Prisms are used clinically to neutralize a deviation between the visual axes of the eyes (in strabismus): the apex of the prism placed before one eye is orientated towards the deviation of that eye; in an esodeviation (e.g. following VI palsy) therefore, the prism is orientated base-out. The strength of Δ incorporated in the spherocylindrical spectacle correction is normally divided equally between the two eyes.

They are also used to measure the angle of deviation in strabismus (Maddox rod test, prism cover test), to assess the stability of binocular fusion (20Δ prism test), and to reveal microtropia (4Δ prism test).

Prisms are also used extensively in optical instruments, which exploit their power to deviate rays without distortion, or invert an image by total internal reflection between the two adjacent surfaces of a right-angle prism.

Fresnel prisms and lenses (Fig. 13.9)

Only the anterior and posterior surfaces of a lens or prism refract light rays; elimination of its centre has no effect on the path of emerging rays. Fresnel lenses and prisms are divided into sections in which the two refracting surfaces are unchanged, but the substance of the intervening lens or prism is minimized, reducing its mass. Plastic Fresnel prisms are applied to spectacle lenses during the period of changing ocular alignment in paralytic squint to prevent diplopia; they can easily be changed as the angle of the squint changes.

The refraction of the eye

The anterior corneal surface produces most of the eye's refracting power, and the aqueous/lens and lens/vitreous interfaces provide variable (in the pre-

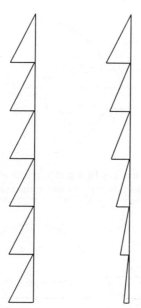

Fig. 13.9   Fresnel prism, and Fresnel lens.

presbyopic eye) additional convergence of light rays. The position of the principal focus of an eye in relation to the retina describes the 'refraction' of the eye.

- In emmetropia the principal focus is on the plane of the retina Fig. 13.10).
- In myopia the principal focus is anterior to the retina (Fig. 13.11).
- In hypermetropia the principal focus is behind the retina (Fig. 13.12), and is therefore virtual.
- In regular astigmatism the eye's refractive power is greatest in one axis, and least at an axis at 90° to this. Lines orientated in both axes cannot be brought to a single focus in one plane (Fig. 13.13).

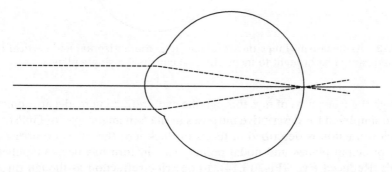

Fig. 13.10   Emmetropia. Parallel rays are brought to a focus at the retinal plane.

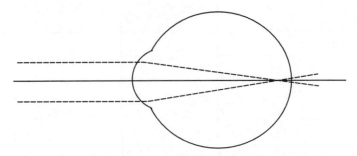

Fig. 13.11   Myopia. Parallel rays are brought to a focus anterior to the retinal plane. Diverging rays (from a near object) form a focus on the retina without accommodation.

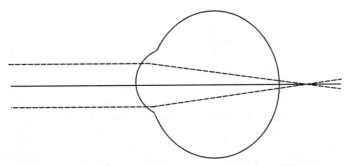

Fig. 13.12   Hypermetropia. Parallel rays are brought to a virtual focus behind the retinal plane. The eye must accommodate to form a real image on the retina.

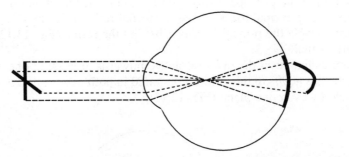

Fig. 13.13   Astigmatism. Lines in two planes (e.g. the horizontal and vertical lines of a cross) cannot be brought to focus simultaneously at a single plane.

Though the true paths of rays through the eye's refracting media are complex, they are simplified for descriptive purposes in the 'schematic eye' of Gullstrand, in which refraction is described in terms of thick lens theory as occurring at a pair of principal planes and nodal points. This in turn has been simplified in Listing's 'Reduced Eye' (Fig. 13.14), to describe refraction as though through a single principal plane *H* and nodal point *N*.

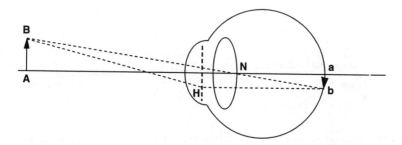

Fig. 13.14   Listing's 'Reduced Eye'. H = single principal plane; N = nodal point.

Clinical refraction

In clinical practice, refraction refers specifically to the measurement of the focusing error (ametropia) of an eye, i.e. the power and sign of lens required to render it emmetropic.

Since image resolution and visual acuity depend upon the focus of the retinal image, it is important to be able accurately to correct the focus of an ametropic eye. The effect on vision of ocular disease can only be accurately assessed when any ametropic error has been corrected, and the ophthalmologist must be able to prescribe spectacles which accurately correct refractive error in order to maximize visual acuity.

Refraction is carried out in two stages:

1. *Objective refraction.* Retinoscopy is used to find the combination of spherical lenses (dioptres sphere, DS) and cylindrical lenses (dioptres cylinder, DC) which neutralize the retinoscopy reflex in the pupil.

2. *Subjective refraction.* The combination of lenses found by objective refraction is placed in a trial frame, and their power and axis are adjusted according to the subject's response, to produce the best visual acuity.

Objective refraction

Retinoscopy

The following description refers to retinoscopy using a streak retinoscope, refracting with spheres. The procedure differs slightly, but the principle remains the same, if a spot retinoscope is used, or if refracting in spheres and cylinders.

With the focusing slide at its lowermost position the retinoscope produces a divergent beam which enters the pupil and illuminates a patch of retina. If the retinoscope is tilted slightly, the illuminated patch of retina moves in the same direction as the movement of the illuminating beam (Fig. 13.15). The refractionist sees the image of the illuminated patch through the pupil. Its position, and the direction of its movement, depend on whether the eye is myopic, emmetropic, or hypermetropic.

Accommodation is prevented by 'fogging' the other eye with a plus lens,

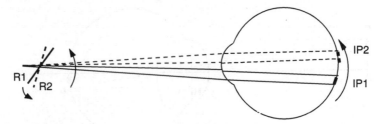

Fig. 13.15   Diverging rays from the retinoscope R1 illuminate a patch of retina IP1. As the retinoscope is tilted upwards to R2, the illuminated retinal patch moves upwards to IP2.

which renders it myopic. In children this may be unreliable, and retinoscopy is performed under cycloplegia, with cyclopentolate or atropine.

Myopia

In the myopic eye, rays leaving the eye from an illuminated point on the retina converge to produce a focus at a near point (in exactly the same way that rays diverging from a near object are focused by the myopic eye on to the retina). As the illuminated retinal point moves in one direction, its image at the near point (its conjugate focus) moves in the opposite direction, and the retinoscopy reflex is seen to move '*against*' the direction of the illuminating beam (Fig. 13.16).

   Placing concave (*minus*) lenses before the eye causes the focus to recede from the near point; a lens of sufficient minus power to neutralize the myopia makes the converging rays leaving the eye parallel, moving the image to an infinitely distant point in front of the eye. At this point (neutralization), the 'against' movement of the retinoscopy reflex is abolished.

Hypermetropia

In the hypermetropic eye, rays from an illuminated retinal point emerge from the eye diverging as if from a point behind the retina (in exactly the same way as a focused retinal image can only be produced in hypermetropia by rays which are converging, before they enter the eye, as though toward such a virtual focal

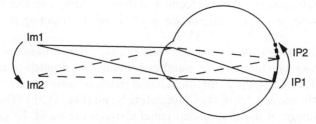

Fig. 13.16   The retinoscopy reflex in myopia. As the illuminated patch moves up, IP2–IP2, its image moves down Im1–Im2. The reflex seen on retinoscopy moves in the opposite direction to ('against') the illuminating beam.

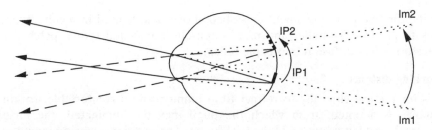

Fig. 13.17 The retinoscopy reflex in hypermetropia. As the illuminated patch moves up, IP1–IP2, its image moves up Im1–Im2. The reflex seen on retinoscopy moves in the same direction as ('with') the illuminating beam.

point). As the illuminated retinal point moves in one direction, its virtual image behind the retina moves in the same direction, and the retinoscopy reflex moves '*with*' the direction of the illuminating beam (Fig 13.17).

Placing convex (*plus*) lenses before the eye reduces the divergence of the emerging rays; a plus lens of sufficient power to neutralize the hypermetropia makes the diverging rays parallel, emerging from a virtual image infinitely distant behind the eye. At this point (neutralization), the 'with' movement of the retinoscopy reflex is abolished.

Astigmatism

The eye's refracting power in one axis is greater than that in an axis perpendicular to it. This is seen on retinoscopy as a movement in one axis while the other is neutralized. A lens of different power is necessary to neutralize each axis.

Emmetropia

Rays from an illuminated retinal point leave the eye parallel, to form an infinitely distant focus (Fig. 13.18). As the retinoscopy beam is moved there is neither with nor against movement of the image: the pupil is fully illuminated when the illuminating beam is axial, and dark when it is not.

If the focusing slide on the retinoscope is moved to its uppermost position, the illuminating beam forms a focus in front of the eye. This causes reversal of

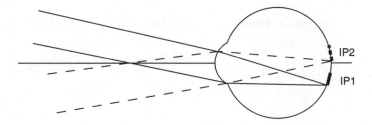

Fig. 13.18 The retinoscopy reflex in emmetropia. The emerging rays are parallel, and the pupil is either illuminated or dark. There is no directional movement of the retinoscopy reflex, since the illuminated patch of retina does not produce an image.

all the directions of movement described above, and is used in highly myopic eyes to produce a smaller and more intensely illuminated retinal patch, and therefore a less diffuse retinoscopic reflex.

Working distance

It is impractical clinically to refract from infinity, and a comfortable working distance is adopted, from which the pupil may be illuminated, the image observed, and lenses placed in the trial frame. The additional converging power required to bring the retinal image from infinity to the refractionist must then be subtracted from the power of lens which neutralizes movement of the reflex.

At a working distance of 1 m, 1DS must be subtracted from the neutralizing lens; at 2/3 m 1.5 DS must be substracted (because the power of a lens is the reciprocal of its focal length), and at 0.5 m 2D must be subtracted. In practice, larger errors occur at shorter working distances, and 2/3–1 m are usually used. Shorter working distances are necessary if media opacities reduce the brightness of the reflex.

To begin it is useful to measure with a tape the precise working distance at which lenses can comfortably be exchanged at arm's length. This distance is automatically adopted with practice, and the allowance necessary is constant and reliably known.

Recording retinoscopy findings (Fig. 13.19)

Draw the lines of a cross to show the direction of movement of the retinoscopy beam, and record the power of the lens which produced neutralization in that direction of movement on each limb of the cross.

Calculating the objective refraction

Subtract the working distance in dioptres algebraically (i.e. with regard to the + or − sign) from the more minus neutralizing lens. This represents the sphere of the objective refraction, and is written above the line as a numerator. Now write the difference between the lens powers in each axis below the line; this is the additional power required to neutralize in that direction of movement, and is the plus cylinder. The axis of the cylinder is the axis in which it has no power; it is perpendicular to its direction of action on the retinoscopy cross.

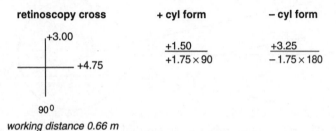

Fig. 13.19 Recording retinoscopy findings, calculating the objective refraction, and transposition.

Transposition

The above descriptions are worked according to the 'plus cylinder' convention; the same spherocylindric refraction may be equally expressed in 'minus-cylinder' form, by altering the spherical power and changing the sign of the cylinder, by a process called 'transposition'. To transpose the sign convention of a sphero-cylindric lens:

1. Calculate the sphere by adding the sphere and the cylinder algebraically (i.e. respecting the + or − signs).
2. Reverse the sign of the cylinder (+ to −, or − to +), and change its axis through 90°.

Though either convention is acceptable, and any correction transposed from one convention to the other is identical, the refractionist is advised to adopt one convention or the other, in order to avoid confusion.

Subjective refraction

The spherical and cylindrical lenses found by retinoscopy are placed in the trial frame. They are adjusted to obtain the best acuity in each eye individually in the following order:

(1) the power of the sphere;
(2) the cylinder axis;
(3) the cylinder power;
(4) the power of the sphere again.

Sphere

Add alternately a +0.5DS and a − 0.5DS to the lenses in the trial frame. Improved acuity with one option or the other indicates either excess − sphere or + sphere, and the trial lenses are adjusted appropriately. Repeat until neither option is preferred

Cylinder

The Jackson's crossed cylinder is a lens with a plus cylinder at 45° to the handle, and a minus cylinder of equal power at 90° to it (and therefore also at 45° to the handle). It is made by grinding a minus cylinder on to a plus sphere of half the power of the cylinder. The axes of the cylinders are marked at the edge of the lens.

The axis of the cylinder in the trial frame is checked by holding the crossed cylinder in front of it, with its axis bisecting those of the crossed cylinder. This is now flipped (rotated in the axis of its handle so that the directions of its + and − axes are reversed), and the acuities in each position are compared. Now rotate the + cylinder in the trial frame towards the + axis of the crossed cylinder in the position in which acuity was better, and repeat the procedure. When the axis is correct, the visual acuities are equal at each flip.

Adjust the power of the trial cylinder in the same way, using the crossed cylinder, but superimpose one axis over that in the trial frame. The flip now increases or decreases the effect of the trial cylinder, indicating whether its power must be increased or decreased to give best acuity.

Duochrome

An overcorrected myopic eye (effectively rendered hypermetropic) can overcome the overcorrection by accommodation. The resulting image is smaller, but may seem clearer because of its higher contrast. The accommodation required to form a focused image becomes uncomfortable, and such an overcorrection is poorly tolerated. The power of the sphere in a myopic correction should be checked using the duochrome test.

Compare acuity to black letters on red and green backgrounds on the duochrome screen. If the letters on green are clearer, the minus correction is too great (Fig. 13.20), and must be reduced until both are equal (Fig. 13.21), or the letters on red are slightly clearer.

The duochrome test works on the principle that the focal plane in the eye of black letters on the green background is anterior to those on the red background, because the shorter wavelength green light is refracted through a greater angle than longer wavelength red light.

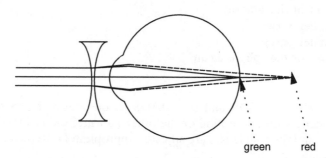

Fig. 13.20 Overcorrected myopia. The image is shifted posteriorly by excess myopic correction, making the most anterior focus (green image) the clearer.

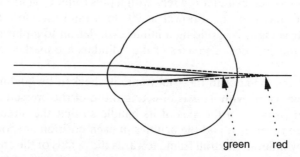

Fig. 13.21 Emmetropia (and accurately corrected myopia). The retinal plane lies between the green and the red focus. The red and green images are equally clear.

Overcorrecting a myope can also be avoided by checking that addition of +0.5DS blurs the best acuity achieved with the proposed correction. If it does not, the proposed myopic correction is excessive.

Presbyopic 'near add'

Presbyopic eyes have a decreased range of accommodation, which can be compensated by the addition of + sphere to the distance correction, to provide reading glasses. These can be dispensed as a separate pair, or as bifocals or varifocals (continuously varying power from the distance correction at the top of the lens to the reading add towards the bottom). Theoretically, the reading addition is calculated to provide some two-thirds of the eye's accommodative reserve. In practice the reading add is often dispensed by rule of thumb, giving 0.5DS at 40–45, and increasing the power incrementally at intervals of about 0.5DS, up to 3.0DS at 65.

Eyes with good distance acuity should manage to read N5 comfortably with an appropriate reading add. Overprescription of the reading add should be avoided by checking that good acuity at arms length (e.g. reading N10) is retained. The appropriate strength of add for near tasks other than reading (e.g. music) can be calculated as the reciprocal of the distance from the eyes to the work.

Recommended further reading

Abrams, J.D. (1993). *Duke–Elder's practice of refraction*, 10th edn. Livingstone, Edinburgh.

Bennett, A.G. and Rabbetts, R.G. (1993). *Clinical visual optics*, 2nd edn. Butterworth-Heinemann, Oxford.

Elkington, A.R. and Frank H.J. (1991). *Clinical optics*, 2nd edn. Blackwell Scientific, Oxford.

Jalie, M. (1980). *The principles of ophthalmic optics*, 3rd edn. The Association of Dispensing Opticians, London.

Michaels, O. D. (1975). *Visual optics and refraction*, 3rd edn. Mosby, St Louis.

14

Lasers in ophthalmology

Principles

Lasers generate light of very high energy by emitting rays of a single wavelength which are coherent (i.e. in phase), and therefore behave like a single 'giant' ray with very high amplitude. The term laser (*Light amplification by stimulated emission of radiation*) describes how coherence and monochromacy are achieved, by pumping energy from a primary source through a medium (gas, crystal, or liquid), which absorbs the energy into its electron orbitals. The energy is emitted in a single wavelength corresponding to the electron energy in the lasing medium, resonates within the medium, and passes through an optical 'valve' which only transmits co-phasic radiation. The wavelength of the emitted laser beam depends on the nature of the lasing medium, and it may be generated in continuous or pulsed form. The wavefront of a pulsed laser may have progressively increasing energy, or be 'Q-switched' to deliver maximum energy instantaneously.

Most surgical lasers use the energy of a laser beam either to disrupt or to photocoagulate tissue. Lasers have particularly useful applications in ophthalmic surgery partly on account of the transparency of the ocular media, which allows direct delivery of the laser energy, and partly because of the relatively low mass of target tissues.

Types of laser

The first ophthalmic lasers (argon) succeeded xenon arc photocoagulators in retinal photocoagulation. Subsequent developments have led to the introduction of: the NdYAG laser (photodisruption and photocoagulation); the diode and the frequency-doubled NdYAG lasers (photocoagulation using solid state lasers); the excimer laser (photoablation); and the HoYAG laser (thermoplasty and thermovaporization).

Laser delivery

Slit-lamp with contact lens

Lasers used for retinal photocoagulation are usually delivered by the slit-lamp through a fundus lens (Volk quadraspheric or area centralis, Rodenstock panfunduscope, or Goldmann 3-mirror). NdYAG laser photodisruption of the iris, posterior capsule or vitreous is also delivered at the slit-lamp, using contact lenses giving high magnification for precise aiming and convergence of the laser beam.

Indirect ophthalmoscope

Argon and diode lasers are available in indirect ophthalmoscope delivery systems, which permit photocoagulation in the supine patient under anaesthetic. This mode is useful in diabetic patients requiring extensive photocoagulation who cannot tolerate treatment at the slit-lamp, and is also useful in the course of vitreoretinal surgical procedures to photocoagulate the margins of retinal breaks.

Endolaser probes

Argon and diode laser can be delivered through an endoprobe in vitreoretinal surgery. The laser beam is transmitted through a flexible fibreoptic cable to a probe introduced into the posterior segment through the pars plana.

Contact probes

A fibre-optic probe with a focusing crystal at its tip, placed at a suitable angle to the axis of the probe, is introduced subconjunctivally to deliver continuous wave NdYAG laser for cyclophotocoagulation, or repetitively pulsed HoYAG laser for photosclerostomy.

Direct delivery with computer-controlled masking

The excimer laser is delivered directly to the cornea in a succession of sweeps of a linear beam, with a mask intervening between laser source and cornea. The profile of the mask is varied under computer control to achieve differential exposure of various parts of the cornea to the photoablative effect of the laser, thereby remodelling the corneal surface.

Table 14.1 shows details of the lasers in current use, their clinical applications, wavelengths, and delivery systems.

Photodisruption

The NdYAG laser emits pulsed infra-red laser radiation (wavelength 1064 nm) from a neodymium-doped yttrium aluminium garnet crystal, in a converging beam which releases all its energy at a very precise focal locus over a period of nanoseconds. The energy density is sufficiently great to cause plasma formation (dissociation of electrons and nuclei), and tissue disruption occurs in the plasma zone. The energy delivered into tissues by the YAG laser is measured in millijoules, and disruption is maximized by Q-switching (delivering maximum energy at once in a square wavefront), and by arranging a rapidly repeating volley of reinforcing shots. Because the NdYAG laser energy is invisible, in the infra-red, clinical delivery systems incorporate a low-energy red helium-neon (HeNe) aiming beam, which is confocal with the YAG.

Photocoagulation

The effect of photocoagulating lasers depends on the local direct and conducted heating effect of energy absorbed by the target tissue. This is determined by the

Table 14.1 Clinical use of ophthalmic lasers

Name	Colour	Wavelength (nm)	Effect	Application	Delivery
Argon	blue green	488 514 530	photocoagulation	diabetic retinopathy SRNVM retinal break trabeculoplasty (ALT)	slit-lamp endo-probe indirect ophthalmoscope
Krypton	red	645	photocoagulation	SRNVM diabetic retinopathy	slit-lamp
Dye	yellow to red	577 to 630	photocoagulation	diabetic retinopathy SRNVM	slit-lamp
Diode	infra-red	810	photocoagulation	diabetic retinopathy retinal break	slit-lamp endo-probe indirect ophthalmoscope
Neodymium YAG NdYAG	infra-red	1064	photodisruption (pulsed mode)	capsulotomy iridotomy	slit-lamp
	infra-red	1064	photocoagulation (continuous wave)	cyclophotocoagulation	slit-lamp contact probe
	green	532	photocoagulation (frequency-doubled continuous wave)	retinal photocoagulation	slit-lamp indirect ophthalmoscope
Holmium YAG HoYAG	infra-red	2100	thermovaporization photothermoplasty	photosclerostomy photothermokeratoplasty	contact probe
Excimer (excited dimer)	UV	193	thermoablation	photokeratectomy photorefractive keratoplasty	direct through mask

wavelength of the laser, target tissue pigment, and the power density of the laser spot. The beam is also absorbed or reflected by pigment in its path, according to the wavelength and the nature of the pigment.

The argon, krypton, and organic dye lasers emit a continuous beam in the visible spectrum, while the diode emits in the invisible infra-red. Exposure time is controlled by an electronic shutter. The variable power is measured in milliwatts, and the beam is focused to concentrate this power into a spot of variable size. The power density therefore increases as the spot-size is reduced, at a given power setting. Having selected a spot-size (50–500 μm) and duration (50–200 ms) appropriate for treatment, power is adjusted to produce the required degree of reaction (normally light blanching). Small spot-sizes (<100 μm) should be avoided, except for direct closure of vessels after pretreatment to whiten surrounding retina, since the high power density in a spot of small size may lead to perforation of Bruch's membrane, and subretinal neovascularization.

Choice of laser wavelength

Table 14.2 shows the wavelengths of emission of ophthalmic photocoagulating lasers, and the absorption maxima of pigments in the eye. Selection of laser wavelength is made by reference to the absorption characteristics of the target tissue, and of adjacent tissue to be spared. In addition, longer wavelengths penetrate lens opacities better than short wavelengths; lower power can be used with less heating of the lens if longer wavelength options are used in eyes with cataract. Recent work suggests that exposure to short wavelength laser may affect cone function, and it is recommended that argon blue is not used.

Therapeutic laser wavelengths for photocoagulation are chosen as follows.

Panretinal photocoagulation (PRP)
- Argon green at 514 nm: maximal absorption by melanin in RPE, and haemoglobin (Hb), with minimal thermal conduction into outer retinal layers.
- Krypton: PRP through vitreous haemorrhage (absorption by melanin in RPE with reduced absorption by Hb in vitreous).

Table 14.2 Wavelengths of ophthalmic lasers and asborption by ocular pigments

---

Laser emission spectra
   argon blue: 488 nm
   argon green: 514 nm
   krypton: 645 nm
   organic dye: variable band from 577 to 630 nm

Pigment absorption spectra
   Hb *maximum at* 550–560 nm
   melanin *maximum at* 550 nm
   xanthophyll *maximum at* 470 nm

Focal macular photocoagulation
- Argon green at 514 nm: maximal absorption by Hb in microaneurysms.
- Dye at yellow 577 nm or orange 590–600 nm: absorption by Hb and melanin, with minimal absorption by xanthophyll.

Photocoagulation of subretinal neovascular membranes
- Krypton red at 647 nm, dye red at 610–633: minimal local macular heating, due to low absorption of energy by Hb.
- Dye at yellow 577 nm or orange 590–600 nm: absorption by pigment in choroid with minimal absorption by macular xanthophyll.

Argon laser trabeculoplasty
Argon green at 514: maximal absorption by melanin.

Surround treatment to retinal breaks
Argon green at 514: maximal absorption by melanin.

Clinical photodisruption

A HeNe red aiming beam is incorporated into the laser, because YAG laser radiation is outside the visible spectrum.

YAG laser capsulotomy

Posterior capsule opacification following extracapsular cataract extraction or phacoemulsification which reduces vision significantly is treated by creating an opening in the axial zone of the posterior capsule with a contiguous series of perforations. Focus the aiming beam on to or slightly behind the capsule, away from the visual axis, through a suitable contact lens. Begin at low energy, increasing as necessary to produce a capsulotomy. Join five to 10 capsulotomies around the visual axis, to provide a clear central gap.

- Use the lowest energy which is effective.
- A 'pulse train' of two shots maximizes the effect of low energy pulses.
- Avoid shots in the intraocular lens (IOL), aiming slightly behind the posterior capsule or selecting the offset function.
- Avoid the central axis (in case of accidental IOL damage).

Record the total energy used, and give acetazolamide s.r. 250 mg, b.d. for 2 days, and topical steroid t.d.s. for 5 days.

YAG laser iridotomy

Pupil block associated with iris bombé is relieved by perforating the peripheral iris in at least two sites. It may be necessary to clear the cornea with intravenous acetazolamide or topical glycerine. Choose the bases of iris crypts for the iridotomies, and avoid vessels and the corneal endothelium. Effective iridotomy is indicated by a fountain of pigment streaming into the anterior chamber as aqueous passes from the posterior to the anterior chamber, and by deepening of the anterior chamber. It is possible to create a partial thickness iridotomy which transilluminates without opening the posterior epithelium fully.

It is important to follow patients with narrow angles, since small YAG iridotomies may undergo delayed closure.

Clinical photocoagulation

Photocoagulation has three therapeutic effects: to ablate ischaemic areas of retina in order to reduce the stimulus to neovascularization; to close subretinal new vessels directly; or to stimulate adhesion of the outer retina to RPE. These three therapeutic intentions are used typically to treat diabetic retinopathy, parafoveal subretinal neovascularization (age-related macular degeneration), and flat retinal breaks, respectively.

When proposing laser treatment it is important to explain to the patient the intention of treatment, and its likely effect on vision. In most cases photocoagulation does not improve vision, but is intended to prevent complications which may impair it. PRP usually causes visual reduction for several hours after treatment, probably on account of dazzle. Visual reduction lasting for up to 3 or 4 weeks may be caused by macular, and sometimes choroidal, oedema. These possibilities should be made clear to the patient before treatment.

Photocoagulation can irreversibly reduce acuity if the fovea is involved in a burn, and great care must be taken to avoid this. The risk is particularly great when using inverting contact lenses (quadraspheric, panfunduscope), and in focal macular treatment—when the beam should only be directed close to the centre if steady fixation is assured, either by good cooperation or akinesia achieved by retrobulbar anaesthesia.

Panretinal photocoagulation

PRP is indicated in retinal neovascular proliferation, or in pre-proliferation if proliferation seems inevitable. Diabetic retinopathy is the commonest cause of neovascularization, but it occurs also following retinal vein occlusion (central and branch), chronic ocular ischaemia ('slow flow' retinopathy in hyperviscosity syndromes and arteriopathy), and sickle cell retinopathy. Generally, the clinical signs are sufficient to identify active fibrovascular proliferation, but fluorescein angiography can help identify areas of retinal ischaemia (as capillary non-perfusion).

The aim of PRP is to reduce the mass of ischaemic tissue, and the oxygen requirement of the compromised retina, until the neovascular stimulus is eliminated. Treatment is easiest at low power slit-lamp magnification, with wide but dim illumination. Retrobulbar anaesthesia can allow much more treatment to be given in fewer sessions, since some patients experience considerable discomfort during PRP, and appreciate fewer sessions and less pain. Alternatively, the treatment may be applied using the indirect ophthalmoscope laser delivery system under general anaesthetic.

Treat in stages of about 1000 burns per session (Fig. 14.1a–e), beginning outside the temporal arcade and on the nasal retina. Use a 500 μm spot-size at 0.2 s, at sufficient power to produce visible blanching (begin at 400 mW for 500 μm spot-size and increase or decrease the power to achieve the correct intensity of

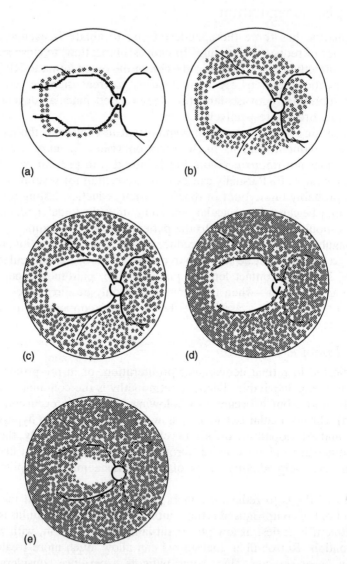

Fig. 14.1 Progressive stages of panretinal photocoagulation (treatment is continued according to this scheme until new vessels have regressed). (a) Initial burns to 'fence off' the macula. (b) Equatorial treatment. (c) Peripheral treatment. (d) Infill. (e) Perimacular treatment.

burn), and separate each burn by 500 μm of untreated retina. Place a 'fence' temporal to the macula, to mark the central limit of temporal PRP (Fig. 14.1a). The Rodenstock panfundoscope and Quadraspheric lenses can be used to place 2000–4000 burns; pre-equatorial treatment usually requires a three-mirror lens. If more than about 4000 burns are necessary, the treated area must be 'filled in' (Fig. 14.1d), and the pre-equatorial and central retina included. Treat within the arcades only if proliferation persists after equatorial and peripheral treatment has been completed, using 200 μm spot-size, and avoid the macula (Fig. 14.1e).

The results of treatment are assessed by the response of the neovascular membranes. Neovascular regression occurs within a few weeks of PRP, and follow up should be arranged to permit further treatment until regression is complete.

Sector PRP is used in branch vein occlusion with signs of ischaemia. It is important to distinguish between new vessels and collaterals in branch retinal vein occlusion (see Chapter 4, p. 61), and not to try to close collaterals.

Focal macular photocoagulation

Diabetic maculopathy occurs in focal exudative, diffuse, and ischaemic forms. Focal exudative diabetic maculopathy responds best to treatment, while ischaemic maculopathy cannot usefully be treated with the laser. Identify focal macular leaks clinically, and if necessary with the help of fundus fluorescein angiography (FFA). 'Treatable macular lesions' are defined in Table 14.3. These are closed directly using 100 μm spot-size at 0.1 s (begin at 80–100 mW). If focal leaks cannot be identified (diffuse maculopathy), treat with a grid of some 100–200 light burns scattered over the extrafoveal macula.

Steady fixation by the patient is very important during macular photo-coagulation, to avoid accidental foveal burn. Ask the patient to fixate a target with the other eye, in order that both eyes are kept still, and use the slit-lamp at high magnification. Avoid treatment in the foveal avascular zone (FAZ = 200 μm, or the thickness of a retinal vein at the disc edge, around the foveola).

Treatment of subretinal neovascular membrane (SRNVM)

Serous elevation at the macula, associated with drusen, localized hard exudates and subretinal haemorrhage, indicates subretinal neovascularization. FFA

Table 14.3   Treatable macular lesions

Microaneurysms >500 μm from the foveola causing thickening (oedema) or hard exudates.

Focal leaks 300–500 μm from the foveola, causing thickening or hard exudate, if visual acuity <6/12, previous treatment has failed to reduce thickening/exudate, and it is judged that treatment will not destroy the perifoveal capillary network.

Areas of diffuse leakage (for grid treatment).

Thickened avascular retina, excluding the FAZ (shown by FFA).

shows early central hyperfluorescence, which increases in size, may have a 'lacey' appearance, and causes late staining. SRNVMs are classified according to their relationship with the FAZ as subfoveal (including the FAZ), juxtafoveal (including the edge of the FAZ), and extrafoveal (entirely outside the FAZ). Extrafoveal SRNVMs are considered treatable if there is a clear margin of retina separating the subretinal membrane from the FAZ.

Direct closure of an extrafoveal SRNVM, together with 100 μm surrounding clear margin, significantly improves the visual prognosis. Repeat FFA 2 weeks following treatment to confirm that closure is complete. Central vision is compromised if SRNVM involving the FAZ is treated, but it is reported that visual prognosis is improved following treatment of central membranes when central vision has already been damaged.

Argon laser trabeculoplasty (ALT)

Very small (50 μm spot-size) burns of high power (750–1000 mW, 0.1 s) are placed on the anterior trabecular meshwork around 180° of the angle, through a gonioprism at high slit-lamp magnification. This treatment reduces IOP by a few mmHg in some patients with POAG. It has no place in the treatment of angle closure or secondary glaucoma. Immediately following treatment the IOP may rise, as a result of trabeculitis; the effects of this may be avoided by a short course of acetazolamide and topical steroid. The IOP-lowering effect of ALT is lost in a proportion of patients after 3 years.

Retinal tears

Flat retinal tears without traction can be surrounded by photocoagulation to stimulate a reactive cellular response, which promotes adhesion between neuroretina and RPE. The break must be surrounded completely by three overlapping rows of overlapping burns, spot-size 500 μm, 0.2 s duration, of sufficient intensity to produce whitening. Breaks with elevated margins, rolled posterior edges, or within retina elevated by subretinal fluid, are not suitable for treatment by photocoagulation alone, and require tamponade.

Clinical photoablation

The excimer laser has recently been introduced as a means of altering the surface contour of the cornea by photoablation. The energy in the ultraviolet radiation is of a frequency which separates intermolecular bonds. Its penetration is low and uniform, so that a single pass across the cornea by an excimer laser beam causes ablation of a precisely controlled thickness of the corneal surface. The corneal epithelium is removed before treatment, and becomes re-established within 2 or 3 days after treatment.

Therapeutic photoablative keratoplasty

The excimer laser is highly effective in removing a thin superficial lamella of corneal stroma, leaving a regular surface for epithelial re-growth. Clinical indications for this therapy include removal of calcium deposits in band kerato-pathy, and superficial corneal scars.

Photorefractive keratoplasty (PRK)

PRK is a form of refractive surgery in which the radius of curvature of the anterior corneal surface is revised in ametropic eyes in order to reduce their refractive error. A computer-controlled mask is programmed to expose different zones of the cornea to different quantities of laser radiation, in order to achieve the desired remodelling effect. Early instruments were designed to treat myopia by flattening the corneal apex; the aperture of an iris diaphragm was reduced progressively, thereby exposing the central cornea to more radiation than more peripheral zones. Newer instruments use a more sophisticated masking system to treat hypermetropia and astigmatism.

Most eyes suffer from a degree of glare following treatment, and the long-term effect of PRK remains to be evaluated. In particular, remodelling may occur, reducing the effect of the correction ('regression').

Recommended further reading

L'Esperance, F.A. (1989). *Ophthalmic lasers*, 3rd edn. Mosby, St Louis.

15

Differential diagnosis of ocular and visual symptoms

Visual symptoms

Poor distance acuity

- uncorrected refractive error, especially myopia
- media opacity
- amblyopia   stimulus deprivation
                             anisometropic
                             strabismic
- keratoconus
- optic neuropathy
- maculopathy
- albinism
- nystagmus   congenital
                           acquired
- achromatopsia
- coloboma involving macula or disc
- posterior pathway or cortical disease.

Night blindness (nyctalopia)

- tapetoretinal degenerations,
- nutritional (vitamin A deficiency, dietary/absorptive defect),
- congenital stationary night-blindness (CSNB),
- advanced glaucoma,
- following extensive panretinal photocoagulation,
- juvenile Batten's disease.

Photophobia

- anterior uveitis,
- anterior cortical lens opacity,
- albinism,
- achromatopsia,
- buphthalmos,
- drugs and toxins,
- psychogenic.

Transient monocular visual loss (amaurosis fugax)

- retinal arteriolar embolization: carotid atheroma; other proximal arterio-pathy (aneurysm, AV malformation, stenosis); cardiac arrhythmia
- papilloedema (obscurations last a few seconds)
- giant cell arteritis
- elevated IOP
- accelerated hypertension and eclampsia.

Bilateral transient visual loss

- syncope,
- low output cardiac failure,
- cardiac arrhythmia.

Sudden monocular visual loss

- giant cell arteritis,
- central retinal artery occlusion,
- central retinal vein occlusion,
- vitreous haemorrhage,
- optic neuritis,
- toxic optic neuropathy (methanol, tobacco/alcohol, quinine),
- optic nerve trauma,
- retinal detachment.

Anterior segment

Conjunctivitis

1. *Acute mucopurulent.* (a) Bacterial (i) *Staphylococcus*; (ii) *Haemophilus*. (b) viral.
2. *Chronic mucopurulent*: (a) associated lid/lacrimal infection; (b) ectropion or entropion; (c) allergic; (d) toxic—topical medication/preservative; (e) other toxic/irritative agents; (f) Reiter's syndrome; (g) gonorrhea.
3. *Ulcerative*: mucous membrane pemphigoid.
4. *Papillary.* Papillae are foci of inflamed hypertrophic tarsal conjunctiva. They are usually smaller and pinker than follicles, and are vascular, the vessels radiating from a central vascular core. They occur in acute inflammation; (a) infective; (b) allergic; (c) toxic.
5. *Follicular.* Follicles are subconjunctival foci of proliferating lymphoid tissue, occurring beneath the upper tarsus. They are pale, slightly elevated, and avascular. They occur in chronic conjunctivitis, especially: (a) viral; (b) chlamydial: (c) allergic and vernal.

Table 15.1 Red eye

	Injection	Pain	Cornea	Discharge	Pupil	Vision	IOP
Conjunctivitis	entire conj including tarsal surface	itching foreign body sensation	clear	purulent/mucopurulent	normal	normal	0
Keratitis	most intensely circumcorneal	ache + foreign body sensation	cloudy stain SPK or focal ulcer	purulent	unaffected or miosed	reduced	0 or −
Episcleritis	deep to conj focal	pricking/mild ache	clear	none	normal	normal	0
Scleritis	livid, deep. Individual vessels may not be seen. Often visible only on lid retraction	severe ache	clear	none	normal	normal or reduced by CME or exudative RD	+ 0 −
Anterior uveitis	most intense circumcorneal	aching photophobia	may be dull due to KP	none	miosed or irregular	normal or reduced	− 0 +
Endophthalmitis	throughout	severe	dull	purulent	normal or miosed	reduced	−
Acute glaucoma	most intense circumcorneal	severe	cloudy due to oedema	none	fixed, mid-dilated	reduced+	++
Subconjunctival haemorrhage	haemorrhage not injection. May elevate conjunctiva	none	clear	none	normal	unaffected	0
Caroticocavernous fistula	prominent engorged large vessels	none	clear	none	normal	unaffected	+

conj = conjunctiva; + = raised IOP; 0 = normal IOP; − = decreased IOP.

Giant papillary conjunctivitis (GPC) occurs in contact lens wearers (especially soft and extended wear contact lenses).

Keratitis

Signs

- Early: epithelial loss, cellular infiltrate, limbal injection, anterior uveitis.
- Intermediate: corneal neovascularization.
- Chronic: fibrous scarring, lipid deposition.

Aetiology

• infection	viral: herpes simplex, zoster
	bacterial: especially *Pseudomonas*, Gram positive cocci fungi: *Asperigillus, Fusarium, Candida*
	protozoa: acanthamoeba
• chemical	caustic alkali
• inflammatory	rheumatoid, Wegener's granulomatosis
• neurotrophic	herpes (zoster, simplex) or V nerve lesion, especially cerebello-pontine angle tumour or post-surgical

Corneal oedema

Corneal oedema is caused by decompensation of the endothelial pump which keeps the stroma in a state of relative dehydration. It may be due to increased hydration pressure or decreased endothelial activity:

• elevated IOP	acute glaucoma
	buphthalmos
	Posner–Schlossman syndrome
• endothelial decompensation	Fuchs' endothelial dystrophy
	post-surgical bullous keratopathy: aphakic; pseudophakic
	anterior segment necrosis
	decompensated keratoconus
	disciform keratitis (focal HSV endotheliitis)
	trauma (tears in Descemet's membrane)
	severe anterior uveitis, especially HSV and HZ
	graft rejection
	iridocorneal endothelial (ICE) syndrome.

Band keratopathy

• chronic inflammation	uveitis and keratitis
• chronic trauma	irritants and trichiasis

- hypercalcaemia   hyperparathyroidism
                          sarcoid
                          renal failure.

Hyphaema

- trauma   closed
                  penetrating
- post-surgical   UGH (uveitis glaucoma hyphaema) syndrome following
                  anterior chamber IOL implantation
- tumours   retinoblastoma
                  iris tumours
- juvenile xanthogranuloma.

Rubeosis

- diabetic retinopathy,
- central retinal vein occlusion,
- chronic ocular ischaemia,
- sickle cell disease,
- chronic total retinal detachment,
- absolute glaucoma,
- intraocular tumour.

Heterochromia

- congenital,
- congenital or infantile Horner's syndrome,
- Fuchs' heterochromic iridocyclitis,
- siderosis (ferrous IOFB),
- iris naevus,
- iris melanoma,
- iris atrophy,
- Waardenburg's syndrome,
- chronic hyphaema,
- ectropion uveae,
- rubeosis.

Anterior uveitis aetiology

- idiopathic;
- HLA B27: ankylosing spondylitis, Reiter's syndrome;
- Crohn's disease, ulcerative colitis;
- Behçet's disease;
- herpes simplex, zoster;

- juvenile rheumatoid arthritis;
- multiple sclerosis;
- secondary to keratitis;
- granulomatous inflammations   *Toxoplasma*
  TB
  sarcoid
  syphilis
- lens-induced.

Cataract aetiology

Congenital
- idiopathic
- intrauterine infection   *Toxoplasma*
  rubella
  cytomegalovirus
  herpes
- chromosome abnormalities
- metabolic   calcium
  galactose 6 phosphate uridyl transferase deficiency
  galactokinase deficiency
- persistent hyperplastic primary vitreous (PHPV)

Acquired
- idiopathic senile
- diabetes
- trauma   physical
  radiation
- anterior uveitis, especially Fuchs' heterochromia
- longstanding total retinal detachment
- steroid-induced (topical or systemic steroid)
- dermatopathies
- calcium metabolic disorder
- retinitis pigmentosa
- dystrophia myotonica.

Dislocated lens

- congenital,
- hereditary,
- traumatic,
- Marfan's syndrome,
- Weill–Marchesani syndrome,
- homocystinuria,
- spherophakia,
- Treacher Collins syndrome.

Posterior segment

Vitreous haemorrhage

- retinal tear
- proliferative retinopathies   diabetic
  central retinal vein occlusion
  branch retinal vein occlusion
  chronic ocular ischaemia
  Eales' disease
- retinal vasculities (Behçet's disease)
- retinitis (CMV, HSV)
- sickle cell disease
- subretinal neovascular membrane
- von Hippel–Lindau disease (retinal angiomatosis)
- X-linked juvenile retinoschisis
- trauma   penetrating
  IOFB
  closed
- intraocular tumour

Macular oedema

- inflammatory   intermediate uveitis
  posterior uveitis
  anterior uveitis
- diabetic   diabetic maculopathy: focal; diffuse
  following PRP
- vascular occlusion   central retinal vein occlusion
  branch retinal vein occlusion
  macular branch retinal vein occlusion
- subretinal neovascularization
- trauma (commotio retinae)
- hypotony
- topical adrenalin (especially following ICCE)
- postsurgical (following intracapsular cataract extraction = Irvine Gass syndrome)
- radiation.

Cherry-red spot at macula

- central retinal artery occlusion
- sphingolipidoses   Tay–Sachs disease
  Niemann–Pick disease
  Gaucher's disease
  infantile metachromatic leucodystrophy

- sialidosis (cherry-red spot—myoclonus syndrome)
- Hurler's syndrome

Bull's eye maculopathy

- toxic: chloroquine, hydroxychloroquine,
- cone dystrophy,
- Stargardt's disease,
- Batten's disease,
- inherited annular macular dystrophy.

Engorged retinal veins

- central retinal vein occlusion
- diabetes
- hyperviscosity states   polycythaemia
                           multiple myeloma
                           macroglobulinaemia
- leukaemia
- lymphoma
- sickle cell disease
- caroticocavernous fistula
- cavernous sinus thrombosis
- congenital AV anomaly.

Retinal neovascularization

- diabetic retinopathy
- retinal vein occlusion   central
                           branch
- chronic ocular ischaemia   hyperviscosity syndromes
                              proximal arterial stenosis
- sickle cell disease
- Eales' disease

Cotton wool spots—focal superficial retinal ischaemia

- systemic vascular   accelerated hypertension
                      eclampsia
                      chronic ocular ischaemia
                      severe hypotension
                      renal disease
- diabetic retinopathy   pre-proliferative
                         proliferative

- inflammatory   collagen vascular disorders: SLE; PAN; severe rheumatoid
                  Behçet's disease
- haematological anaemia
                  leukaemia
                  myeloma
                  Hodgkin's disease
- infective   AIDS
                  CMV
                  HSV (acute retinal necrosis)
                  subacute bacterial endocarditis

Angioid streaks

- idiopathic,
- pseudoxanthoma elasticum,
- Ehlers–Danlos syndrome,
- Paget's disease,
- acromegaly.

Choroidal folds

- orbital mass,
- high hypermetropia,
- dysthyroid ophthalmopathy,
- choroidal tumour,
- scleral buckle (after retinal detachment surgery),
- hypotony.

Elevated optic disc

Pathological causes

- papilloedema
- papillitis
- anterior ischaemic optic neuropathy (AION)   cranial arteritis
                                                arteriopathy
                                                accelerated hypertension
- diabetes
- optic disc drusen
- hypotony
- leukaemia
- nerve/disc tumour   meningioma
                       glioma
                       neurofibroma

Non-pathological causes

- hypermetropia,
- Bergmeister's papilla,
- anomalous retinal vessels.

Papilloedema

The term papilloedema refers to optic disc swelling associated with raised CSF pressure. Visual acuity is unaffected, except during characteristic 'obscurations', which last for a few seconds.

Causes of papilloedema

- intracranial tumour obstructing CSF circulation (NB pituitary tumour rarely raises ICP),
- benign intracranial hypertension,
- hydrocephalus,
- cerebral abscess,
- intracranial aneurysm,
- intracranial haemorrhage,
- meningitis and encephalitis,
- optic nerve tumour,
- orbit tumour,
- Paget's disease,

Papillitis

The term papillitis describes disc elevation due to inflammation. Because the optic nerve is inflamed, visual acuity is inevitably reduced, and there is a relative afferent pupil defect.

Causes of papillitis

- demyelination
- vasculitis   PAN
                        SLE
- adjacent inflammation orbit
                        sinus
                        retina
                        choroid
- viral infection   Epstein–Barr
                        CMV
- nutritional
- toxic
- photocoagulation

Ocular motility

Diplopia

Monocular

- Spectacles   improperly centred lenses
                inaccurate cylinder axis
                inappropriate prism
- Eye   irregular astigmatism
                corneal scar
                cataract, especially nuclear sclerosis
                dislocated or ectopic lens
                eccentric IOL
                second pupil (iridectomy, iris atrophy)
                psychogenic

Binocular

- Muscle imbalance   III, IV, VI palsy
                      Postoperative overcorrection (squint surgery)
                      Explant effect (detachment surgery)
                      abnormal retinal correspondence
                      thyroid eye disease
- Other   aniseikonia (high anisometropia, e.g. unilateral aphakia)
                      decompensation of heterophoria
                      psychogenic

Pseudo-extraocular muscle palsies

- myasthenia gravis,
- Duane's lid-retraction syndrome,
- cross-fixation,
- fibrosis of antagonist,
- surgical overcorrection.

Nystagmus

Congenital nystagmus

- Without eye or visual pathway disorder.
- Associated with   albinism,
                   congenital cataract,
                   achromatopsia,
                   Leber's amaurosis and tapetoretinal degeneration,
                   optic nerve hypoplasia,
                   retinal detachment,
                   optic nerve glioma,
                   spasmus nutans.

- Characteristic features   horizontal uniplanar,
  increased on fixation,
  damped on convergence,
  optokinetic nystagmus (OKN) appears reversed,
  null-point determines abnormal head posture.

Acquired nystagmus

- Vestibular   labyrinthine   } constant in all gaze positions
  nuclear
- Central   pontine
  cerebellar   } gaze-evoked
  drug-induced

Demyelinating disease produces both vestibular and gaze-evoked patterns.

Pseudosquint

- epicanthus (skin folds across medial canthi),
- negative angle kappa (temporalization of the visual axis),
- telecanthus (wide separation between medial canthi),
- hypertelorism (widely spaced orbits),
- hypotelorism (closely-spaced orbits),
- other congenital orbital malformations.

Conjugate gaze paresis

* *Frontal cortex*   destructive lesions cause failure of contralateral gaze deviation
  irritative lesions cause temporary unsteady contralateral gaze
  deviation
  reflex gaze deviations are normal.
* *Brainstem*   destructive lesions cause failure of ipsilateral gaze
  irritative lesions cause transient unsteady ipsilateral gaze deviation
  reflex gaze deviations are absent.

† Frontal eye fields (frontal cortex) drive saccades toward the opposite side.
† Horizontal gaze centres (pons) drive gaze deviations to the same side.
† Vertical gaze centre (midbrain) are bilateral.

Reflex stimulation of conjugate gaze deviation

- doll's head,
- rotation (vestibulo-ocular response, VOR),
- OKN (optokinetic nystagmus),
- caloric tests (cold water into external auditory meatus causes ipsilateral gaze
  deviation, and contralaterally-directed nystamgus),
- Bell's phenomenon.

External ophthalmoplegia including ptosis, but sparing pupils

- III palsy,
- myasthenia,
- chronic progressive external ophthalmoplegia (CPEO)
- ophthalmoplegia plus (CPEO + pigmentary retinopathy and cardiac abnormalities),
- Steel–Richardson syndrome,
- Guillain–Barré and Miller–Fisher syndromes,
- motor neurone disease.

Complete ophthalmoplegia involving pupils

- demyelinating disease,
- brainstem infarct,
- aneurysm,
- cerebello-pontine angle tumour,
- encephalitis,
- head injury.

Painful ophthalmoplegia

- diabetes,
- hypertension and arteriosclerosis,
- tumour,
- intracavernous aneurysm of internal carotid artery,
- orbital inflammation,
- orbital cellulitis and abscess,
- cavernous sinus thrombosis,
- ophthalmoplegic migraine,
- orbital malignancy.

Neuro-ophthalmology

III, IV, and VI palsies

Pathology may be in the:

- nucleus or intracerebral fascicle;
- intracranial, intracavernous/superior orbital fissure or orbital course of the nerve.

III, IV, and VI are all vulnerable to:

- *nucleus, fascicle, intracranial*   ischaemia (diabetes, hypertension, thrombosis, embolus, giant cell arteritis)

demyelination
tumour (primary, metastatic)
compression (aneurysm, tumour)
inflammation (meningitis, encephalitis)
Guillain–Barré/Miller–Fisher syndrome
amyotrophic lateral sclerosis
trauma

- *cavernous sinus, superior orbital fissure*
  aneurysm
  meningioma
  pituitary tumour
  craniopharyngioma
  nasopharyngeal tumour
  metastasis
  infection/inflammation

- *orbit (orbital III lesions affect single muscles or muscle groups)*
  inflammation
  ischaemia
  infiltration
  compression
  trauma

Specific causes of lesions of III, IV, VI

- III aneurysm
  posterior communicating artery
  posterior cerebral artery
  basilar artery
- IV congenital
  trauma
- VI aneurysm
  ant inf cerebellar artery
  post inf cerebellar artery
  basilar artery
  internal carotid artery (cavernous sinus)

  trauma
  raised intracranial pressure
  acoustic neuroma
  mastoiditis (Gradenigo's syndrome)

Anisocoria

One to 2 mm anisocoria in 20 per cent of normals.

Small pupil

- physiological miosis,
- senile
- Horner's syndrome,
- miotics,

- anterior uveitis,
- posterior synaechiae,
- aphakia,
- dislocated lens,
- anaesthesia and coma,
- meningitis, encephalitis,
- histaminic cephalgia,
- Argyll Robertson pupil,
- drugs.

Large pupil

- physiological mydriasis
- III palsy
- Adie's myotonic pupil
- pharmacological   cholinergic blockers
                                 adrenergic agonists
- iris atrophy   ischaemic
                                 herpes simplex kerato-uveitis
- acute glaucoma
- IOFB
- photocoagulation
- aniridia
- coma

Relative afferent pupil defect (RAPD)

- optic neuropathy   ischaemic
                                 demyelinating
                                 inflammatory
                                 tumour
                                 toxic
- retinal detachment
- advanced glaucoma
- extensive panretinal photocoagulation
- advanced myopic degeneration

Optic neuropathy aetiology

- *papillitis*: inflammatory signs at elevated optic disc, reduced acuity;
- *retrobulbar neuritis*: no abnormal ophthalmoscopic signs.

Aetiology

- demyelinating   single isolated episode, or part of MS
                                                             transverse opticomyelitis (Devic's)

- anterior ischaemic optic neuropathy   giant cell arteritis
  arteriosclerosis
  arterial embolus
  accelerated hypertension
- hereditary optic atrophy   Leber's optic atrophy
  dominant optic atrophy
- orbital inflammation: HZO, abscess, sinusitis
- meningitis and encephalitis
- following viral illness (especially in children)
- adjacent chorioretinitis
- Behçet's disease
- leukaemia
- metabolic   diabetes, nutritional (B vitamin deficiency)
- drugs and toxins   tobacco-alcohol amblyopia
- CMV, AIDS

Orbit

Orbital pain

- retrobulbar neuritis,
- orbital cellulitis,
- Tolosa–Hunt and orbital apex syndromes,
- sinusitis,
- dacryoadenitis,
- viral illness,
- ophthalmoplegic migraine,
- asthenopia.

Ptosis

Congenital

- simple congenital,
- congenital Horner's syndrome,
- developmental lid abnormality,
- Marcus–Gunn jaw-winking syndrome,
- aberrant III nerve.

Acquired

- involutional (degenerative weakening of levator aponeurosis)
- neurogenic   III nerve palsy
  Horner's syndrome
  multiple sclerosis
  aberrant III regeneration

- myogenic
  ocular myopathy
  dystrophia myotonica
  myasthenia
- mechanical
  acquired lid abnormality: tumour; inflammation
  cicatricial
  contact lens-associated
- trauma
- following eye surgery
- steroid induced (chronic topical steroid use)

Exophthalmos

Inflammatory

- dysthyroid ophthalmopathy,
- orbit cellulitis or abscess,
- pseudotumour,
- sarcoid.

Neoplastic

Primary benign

- dermoid,
- neurofibromatosis,
- optic nerve glioma,
- optic nerve sheath meningioma,
- sphenoid ridge meningioma extension,
- lacrimal gland tumour,
- juvenile xanthogranuloma.

Primary malignant

- rhabdomyosarcoma,
- malignant lacrimal gland tumour,
- lymphoma,
- histiocytosis X.

Secondary

- leukaemia,
- nasopharyngeal or sinus carcinoma,
- extraocular spread malignant melanoma,
- neuroblastoma (infants),
- lung,
- breast,
- prostate.

Vascular

- haemangioma,

- varices,
- caroticocavernous fistula.

Trauma

- intraorbital foreign body,
- retrobulbar haemorrhage.

Pseudoproptosis

- unilateral myopia,
- buphthalmos,
- megalocornea,
- lagophthalmos,
- contralateral enophthalmos or ptosis,
- craniofacial dysostosis.

Enophthalmos

- senile,
- blowout fracture of orbit,
- cachexia,
- pseudo-enophthalmos: contralateral exophthalmos.

Recommended further reading

Roy, F.H. (1989). *Ocular differential diagnosis*, 4th edn. Lea & Febiger, Philadelphia.

Index